I FOUND MY TRIBE

I FOUND MY TRIBE

Ruth Fitzmaurice

Chatto & Windus
LONDON

1 3 5 7 9 10 8 6 4 2

Chatto & Windus, an imprint of Vintage,
20 Vauxhall Bridge Road,
London SW1V 2SA

Chatto & Windus is part of the Penguin Random House group of companies
whose addresses can be found at global.penguinrandomhouse.com.

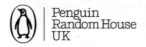

Penguin
Random House
UK

Hand lettering by Lily Jones

First published in the UK by Chatto & Windus in 2017

penguin.co.uk/vintage

A CIP catalogue record for this book is available from the British Library

HB ISBN 9781784741464
TPB ISBN 9781784741471

This book is a work of non-fiction based on the life, experiences and
recollections of the author. In some limited cases the names of people and
details of events have been changed solely to protect the privacy of others.

Typeset in 10/18 pt MillerText
By Jouve (UK), Milton Keynes
Printed and bound by Clays Ltd, St Ives plc

Penguin Random House is committed to a sustainable future
for our business, our readers and our planet. This book is made
from Forest Stewardship Council® certified paper.

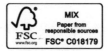

MIX
Paper from
responsible sources
FSC
www.fsc.org   FSC® C018179

For my parents, Pat and Dave O'Neill

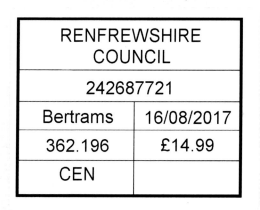

'I must be a mermaid, Rango, I
have no fear of depths and a great
fear of shallow living.'

Anaïs Nin, *The Four-Chambered Heart*

Contents

The Sea

Three-year-old Sadie says that Dadda talks with his eyes. An eye gaze computer sounds less romantic. I'll ask his eyes she says when she wants something. He loves me! she exclaims like a surprise present. Love like a present is the gift we share from him. I hold it fiercely. His magnificent heart.

My husband is a wonder to me but he is hard to find. I search for him in our home. He breathes through a pipe in his throat. He feels everything but cannot move a muscle. I lie on his chest counting mechanical breaths. I hold his hand but he doesn't hold back. His darting eyes are the only windows left. I won't stop searching. My soul demands it and so does his. Simon has motor neurone disease, but that's not the dilemma, at least not today. Be brave.

I am sitting in my car in Wicklow town, looking out on the harbour. I'm watching these yacht masts dancing. Their heads are swaying to and fro, warbling along to Joni Mitchell on the radio.

Wicklow harbour is nice. It's vast and full of blue. It has a higher, wider reach than the Greystones view. I feel as though I can't breathe in Greystones right now, so Wicklow is good. Maybe Greystones is like all great loves. You either marvel at every familiar dancing step and soak it into your bones or, like today, the familiar edges trip you up and annoy the shit out of you. Too claustrophobic – a rat in a cage, a lift with no panic button.

Here's the dilemma. My house is full of strangers. I have painted it bright colours and surrounded it with love, but strangers step through it at an alarming rate. Well-meaning Muhammads make tea. So many Helens and Marys and Jackies and Michaels and Deirdres and Claires and Sams and Franks and Graces smile and leave mops in weird places. I sidestep them in the hall and at the dishwasher. Our house is filled with nurses and carers and they are hurting me. It's not their fault.

Some stay a while, but most are passing through. Some stay longer. I grow to love them and then they break my heart and leave anyway. It's nobody's fault. This is agency work. Some wear overbearing perfume. It attacks olfactory emotions I didn't even know I had. I feel irrational hatred towards them because they make my house smell like *them*. Most of them smoke but I don't mind the smell of that. At least it's a universal smell, like fire or Fairy Liquid or Persil Automatic or petrol. A lot of them try and turn our home into a hospital, and I fight like a tiger against that and bare pointy teeth.

They all leave eventually, except for Marian. Marian believes in angels and blood moons. She lives purely through her emotions, and a good day always starts with this night nurse. We drink tea together on dark mornings. I wish I believed in angels. Marian believes everything happens for a reason and that people have colours and swirling energy around them, positive or negative.

If you hang out with her for long enough, you could be laughing or crying or both and you can almost see a faint outline on the walls of angel wings in the shadows. She is, of course, my angel. 'I'm not going anywhere,' she said to me once. 'I'm here for you.' I look into her eyes and I believe her.

There was a blood moon last night and the sea is agitated. My soul is agitated. The full moon gets a red glow during a lunar eclipse, says Marian, so watch out. Blood moons belong to moongazers, dreamers and to Marian. For them, the night sky is a realm of intense feeling and romance. I'd never heard of such things, so I lean in closer. We are up to eighty per cent water, Marian says, and that is why the moon and the tides affect us. That is why I jump in the sea, I say. I am trying to find a home, make a home, *be* a home for my five children. Sometimes I succeed and sometimes I fail.

*

Some people understand that the small things make a difference. A nice pen to write with that slides perfectly on the page. Hot coffee in a particular cup. These things matter when your soul is on the edge. It fills you full of holes, this life. My search for Simon is a lonely pursuit. I hope he looks for me too. Great love has brought me to the sea and I am trying to be brave. It's important, when your soul just might need saving.

We have lost many things. But sometimes I find my husband: lips on the curve of his temple, a crawl space in the crook of his arm. Some things are lost and found again. I email him words of love, and he emails back. A mad moon tidal wave. Screen to screen, we're holding hands at last. Two souls. It's a marvellous, familiar dance. Great loves are for the brave.

My Cove

I have to tell you a secret. This is my cove. No really, it's actually mine. So says an old lady who rolls up on a flowery purple pushbike one day. We are standing in swimming hats, my friends and I. Three women at Ladies' Cove, the steps that lead into the sea at Greystones, Co. Wicklow. We are standing, turning slightly blue on a sunny April day. The air is warm but those in the secret all-year swim club know that the sun is deceptive. The sea is bloody freezing at this time of year. Colder than Christmas.

We are trying to be brave. It's my cove, says the old lady, as she hitches a foot to the ground, leaning her purple bike into a chat. We don't want to chat, we want to dive, but she isn't going anywhere. She is lonely and wants to talk to us and that's that. I aspire to be this old lady some day. I would feel lucky to grow old like her, on her flowery bike, wind in her hair, stopping to chat when she feels like it and when she needs it. Some old ladies are great like that. I aspire to be her because, obviously, it's not her cove at all. It's mine.

I collect stones on the beach. My favourites are the grey ones full of holes. The sea made these holes; each one is different and beautiful. I rattle them home in my pocket and arrange them on windowsills.

My swimming friend has a cousin who is one of those calm people who are healing to be around. A cup of tea with her in summer garden sunshine reveals to me that I am not a calm person. I yearn for her serenity. We were talking about a first-world problem, maybe a universal problem: the dilemma of where to live.

We have love in the nucleus of our family, but where do you put roots down with that love? An affordable bigger house in the countryside, or a commutable distant town? Or stay where you know people, in a smaller house bursting at the seams? My friend's calm cousin cuts through the bullshit. 'Find your tribe,' she says. Finding your people is more important than what kind of house you live in. Decide whether you've found your tribe and go from there. I believe her.

The cove is my tribe and the cove is mine. My babies stand with soggy shoes on the shore, skidding on wet stones and cheer as their Momma plunges to her salvation. Yes, this is my cove and the sea is my salvation. It shocks my body back to life, as rain darts on the sea surface on a misty, romantic day.

On other days I need to weep. When your body breaks down in a parked car, it is embarrassing. A man walked by on the footpath at the precise moment my face crumbled, and I turned away sharply. Oh, the shame. The horror that someone should witness this pain in the safe routine of the school run.

On this day I can't escape the feeling of being in a ransacked house full of strangers. I cry for all the things we have lost, my husband and I. I thought of stepping out of the car in the rain. Step out and walk in the rain to the sea, to the steps down to the cove. To just step into the waters and struggle in my winter jacket and not come back up.

I could never do that because of the five snoring beauties at home. My five beautiful children. Jack, age ten, still has cheeks like velvet. Eight-year-old Raife looks uncannily like his father. At seven, Arden is a whirlwind spinning his own way. There is nothing final about four–year-old twins. Hunter's green eyes startle me daily. The sweep of Sadie's curls are the closest I've come to a God.

Some people took over our cove one day, a group of tourists who announced they were jumping in with their clothes on. I stared at this lady in horror, with her big winter coat, and remembered I had thought of jumping in myself not so long ago. But this was no tragic, Virginia Woolf, stones-in-her-pockets endeavour. They were whooping and laughing.

'Are they drunk?' I muttered to my swimming friend.

'No, I think they're just American,' she said honestly, and we both got a fit of the giggles. They rolled up like happy doughnuts from the YMCA. A religious cleansing? I kept eyeing the American woman's puffy winter jacket and imagined her swirling under with the seaweed. They marched in from the shore, arms raised in triumph, and emerged John-the-Baptist-style.

But on another day I stood at the edge of the sea and wept. My feet were submerged on the bottom step and I wiggled my red toenails and sobbed. My sea-swimming friend was there to hug me. The sea was choppier but my soul was calmer and refreshed and content when I climbed back up the steps. We may be eighty per cent water, Marian, I think, but my emotions are as mysterious to me as the swell of the sea. All I know is that I could never leave this place. The cove is my tribe and the sea saves me.

We all gather here at the cove: the lost, the happy, the lonely, the young. The old lady on her purple bike, a bride posing for photos in blue sparkly shoes. So many walkers and thinkers with labradoodles, poodles, bichons and pugaliers. A lady collects sea glass on the shores every morning marching in time to the beat from her earphones. A group huddles to smoke cigarettes. Toddlers laugh and chase waves. Dogs bark. Men fish. And some of us swim. In summer, teenagers squeal at the cold and make boastful jumps from high rocks. In autumn, hardy wrinkled old-timers pace their breast stroke. But most of the year it's just me. I'm alone at my cove and it's mine. Come join me for a visit. Dive in for a swim. Be brave. But just remember this is *my* cove. No really. It's mine.

Michelle

A group of renegades gather at Greystones harbour on 14 September 2014. The new marina at the harbour is a grey pillared beast left half unfinished. A slipway slides boats straight into the water and out to sea. This group hasn't gathered for a boat, but for a man called Galen. He has struggled into a wetsuit in cold September. Two Trojan helpers join hands to give him a king's chair lift to the slipway and slide him in. His legs are paralysed, but a gruelling regime has made his arms super-strong. He harnesses his lower half into motion with these arms and swims like a gently swirling fish out of the mouth of the beast and way out to sea.

My local hairdresser is a girl with kind eyes. She charms me with genuine chat that chimes like a bell. I've sat in her salon several times now. She always laughs and greets me as the crazy lady with five children. But she doesn't know about

Simon. I worry about people. I tend not to tell them about MND, especially hairdressers. The shock might hurt them and they are holding scissors.

But my mood is bubbly today and then, magically, Simon and MND spill out. The scissors freeze in her hand and I see her take a breath. 'You know,' she whispers, 'you really remind me of another lady who comes in here. Her husband crashed his bike on the N11 and he's in a wheelchair now. Just before it happened she found out she was pregnant with their fourth child. Imagine that! The last possible moment they could have a baby. But this lady? So beautiful! Her smile! She brings the baby in here and he has this long blond hair in a clip. I thought he was a girl, he's so pretty!' I nod and glow with pride. Of course I know. This lady is my friend. Like a conch of whispering sea sounds you hold to your ear in wonder, her name is Michelle. She is my sea swimming buddy.

Six years before, a long time in MND years, Simon and I had a memorable night out. The comedian Tommy Tiernan was ranting and raving onstage with pure abandon. Simon's immobile legs meant he was wheelchair bound back then, but his upper body was still unaffected. He laughed and talked along with everyone else. He held my hand. Tommy's euphoric eyes are wild windows into happy madness. He turned his gaze on the wheelchair section. 'Howya. You lads in the wheelchairs,' he growled. 'The ANGER comin' off ya.

The POWER of it. FUCK, it's like a car battery.' Simon howled with laughter.

Swimming at the marina is just not allowed because of the boats, but today, we allow ourselves to be renegades. Children skip over stones, mothers sway buggies, men put out picnic blankets and packets of crisps. This is civilised law-breaking to celebrate another man who is like a car battery. We all join him in the water to wave and cheer as he swims out to sea. He makes it all the way around the headland to Ladies' Cove. Galen is Michelle's brave husband. It is a year to the day since his racing bike crashed on the N11.

Greystones encloses a semicircle of sea. Driving down the hill from Bray we salute it. The seafront sweeps walkers into wildness and then back into the heart of the town. Somehow, I have lived in Greystones all this time and avoided the sea. I almost forgot it was there. I have glanced at it and then busied myself with the day.

Galen's car battery has brought me here. His defiance drives me into the water with him and it is bloody freezing. We are all laughing hysterically. Galen disappears around the headland and we gather in our towels, and drink hot whiskeys. Michelle weaves her way through the crowd, new baby on her hip. He is their war baby and she is smiling, but her eyes are haunted. Michelle and Galen used to swim together every day and all year round. Even gloriously pregnant she would hurl herself into the water. Their three older children jump from high rocks, but she stays by the shore looking terribly young.

Galen is swimming out to sea for a reason. He is swimming quite simply to save his soul. When tragedy hits, you need saving. You search for moments to save yourself. I have saved myself so many times I am bloody exhausted. But Galen's tragedy is still fresh. His defiance is electric. Against it, I feel old and weary and tired. Simon is not with us at the marina. He is home in bed engaged in his virtual world. His eye gaze computer doesn't work outdoors and making the trip to the marina is too hard. We have lived with MND for six years and I am jaded.

Simple solitary moments have saved my soul through these MND years. These moments might seem silly to others but they have steadied me. Standing on the slipway, I realise they have all been out of doors.

In daylight hours, a garden bench has saved me. I stole moments from screaming kids on this bench, at our first family home in Co. Louth. Outdoors I gazed at trees with hot coffee in my hands. I spend a lot of my time gazing at trees. In Greystones, the same bench, now painted red, sits out the front, like a beacon, just in case.

Washing lines have saved me. I stole moments of peace in our country garden, hanging washing out, in my wellies. In the heat of Australia, where we holidayed for a while, saving your soul was simpler. The scorched washing line was warm and we had an outdoor swimming pool. On early bright mornings, I wielded a net across the pool for its daily clean, while I danced in my underwear.

On darkest nights the sky has always saved me. In the countryside I would throw open the half-door and stand under the vast starry sky. In Australia, the hot creak of crickets drowned out the darkness. In Greystones, I still creep out the back at night to howl at the moon.

Our pain is not static. It never rests. Galen has channelled his pain out to sea, to find the thing that will save him there. We just want to cope, to exist and to function. We also want to live. Today at the marina it's Galen's moment.

My friend Aifric and I gravitate towards one another. We have been friends a long time. We are both locked into Michelle's pain. We can feel it. We look at each other and nod. Michelle has to get back to swimming. We have no choice but to become her new swimming buddies. No words are needed but Aifric and I are equally petrified.

Galen's bike crash was an instant cut with the cruellest knife. With MND the loss is different. It's a steady crumble. Limbs get weaker. Function dwindles subtly. It's the reverse of a child growing before your eyes. Huddled on the beach post-swim, Michelle and I will debate the differences between these losses. Swaddled in blankets with the sea shakes, we often share a single flask of tea. Which is worse? we will wonder. To lose everything in a moment, or have it gradually taken from you? We won't know the answer but will agree that they are equally shit.

We will do these things because pain never stops. One man's defiance at the marina can change a moment. But a single moment won't save you. We all need saving again and again and again. Galen is not saved on his day at the marina, but the moment of his accident is redefined. Michelle is not saved, nor is Aifric, nor am I. But the Tragic Wives' Swimming Club is formed.

Friends

My very best friend in the world is a tree. Hello, Tree. Tree is a beautiful birch. She sits outside my window. Her boughs rattle in winter and sway in spring. Tree is also a she because I need her to be. We share deep thoughts over coffee. 'Shhh! Momma is talking to her tree!' my five ducklings hiss. They creep in and fold themselves around me but know not to interrupt. I have trained my ducklings well. Daydreaming is a valued skill in our home. Dare to interrupt it. 'Momma, you just broke an important daydream,' Raife, my eight-year-old, will scold. 'Sorry,' I will say, with real regret.

This little house of ours holds a lot. A family of five children, a father who can move only his eyes, a daydreaming mother, a mass of medical equipment that hums and squeaks. The swirly mad vortex of MOTOR NEURONE DISEASE. We are spinning, surviving and trying not to get pulled down the plughole. The footfall is high in this house. I should hoover more. Nurses and carers steer tactful soft shoes around us all. Lint balls gather in corners. My husband needs a ventilator to breathe and a person to stay with him at all times. Often that person is me. I spend a lot of time in this house and Tree really helps.

When I was at school, I was runner-up in an art competition. The Minister for Health gave me a prize for my grey pencil drawing of a sad girl reading a book. Outside her window, a group of children played in full colour. My poster slogan to promote healthy living read, 'Life Is No Fun In The Company Of One'.

Company is not a problem for me these days. I am just so popular in here. How could I ever be lonely in this house? That schoolgirl knew nothing about this life. Raife loves the word 'inappropriate' but I don't think he knows what it means. His use of it is downright inappropriate. 'Don't talk about me to other people,' he scolds, 'it's inappropriate'. It seems that eight is the age of reason. The age a child sees their own nakedness and roars 'Don't see me! Don't judge me!' They scold their mothers often. My own mother sees too much even from the end of a phone. She holds that special mother key. Turn it half an inch and the tears will flow. My mother might be my friend but really she is something else. She is the only person who will ever worry if I leave the house without a coat on.

Simon's MND has made me wildly inappropriate. I have no social filter. I don't remember the rules. I worry about wearing this pain in company. How much is too much? Simple questions like 'How are things?' become impossible. Thank God for old friends. They are like wishing wells; my pain is a stone that won't make a splash. New friends are tricky. Maybe I don't need them? My three-year old is screaming at me because his shadow won't go away. He growls his drunken toddler slur, 'Stupid Momma. Stupid shadow.' These children are everything but they are not my friends. Mostly they're not even friendly. The schoolgirl was right. I am a pencil drawing in grey. I am so popular in here it stinks. Even the dog and the cat agree. I am talking to a tree, for God's sake. I need some colour and company.

Company scares me. I must venture out with armour on. My slogan will be a happy one. So many beautiful women greet me and take me into their company. In the right frame of mind, in the right moment, I am enjoying this. The subtle orchestra of the chit and the chat. I am enjoying it all. Eye-rolls at the mention of the husbands. He never helps. Problems at work. I got him a gym membership for Christmas. I am enjoying this, really am. I just feel a bit tired. I am fighting the urge to just lie down on the ground and cover myself with a blanket. I smile at them all and feel like an alien. Their problems are just as important as mine. How are things? I have no language for this. I will go home to my husband because he is my friend. Eye-roll. He is a friend, he's my very best husband. Don't see me! Don't pity me! Stupid company. Stupid MND.

But company keeps calling and I'm too stubborn to quit. Somewhere above the chit and the chat a woman I barely know announces that her marriage just ended and her husband is living in the shed at the bottom of their garden. The collective clink of coffee cups goes silent. It's a show-stopper. We all mutter condolences. Company is humbled and so am I. And then, blessedly, the chat moves on.

Walking home alone I laugh out loud, not at this woman's pain, but at my own stupidity. The rules were all in my own head. Wear as much pain as you like, or wear none. Stupid rules. Stupid me. I laugh because colour is all around me and company is my new best friend.

Daydreams

I've spent most of my life in a daydream. Ireland can be so cloudy and grey it feels like somebody turned the lights out. Daydreaming really helps with this. Lights don't matter much when your dreams are shiny. Daydreams just don't care if it's cloudy.

Parents perpetuate certain stories about their children that become pure fact. 'You were always a child who loved her bed,' my mother still says. 'You never wandered from it. Once you went in there, you never came back out till morning.' Of course I didn't. Bed is the birthplace of dreams and daydreams. Bed was my safe harbour after steering the dark waters of reality all day.

I spent glad nights and endless daylight hours as a little girl nesting in my bed. Outside of the brightly lit kitchen our house was old and cold and creepy, but I didn't care. From my bed I was too busy staring at my radiator. It had faces on it. Endless fantastical faces, shapes and stories. They leaped out from the warped leaky paint. My radiator was like Lucy's wardrobe. It transported me to Narnia every time.

'Dinnertime!' my mother would call from the warmth of the kitchen. Food is possibly the only acceptable reason to break a daydream. I would leap out of my daydream and in my head I was cheering, 'I'm here! I've come back! It's all right!' Hasn't anyone wondered where I've been? Have seconds or hours or days just passed? But in a big old busy house of six children, nobody had really noticed. Nobody noticing made the daydreams more wonderful.

Daydreams were solitary things until somebody noticed. Simon arrived and interrupted my daydreams. Simon spoke in CAPITAL LETTERS. He sauntered up all blue eyes and dancing hands. His voice strolled right through my daydreams and had a good gawk. He talked a lot and I liked his talk. The Voice and the Daydreamer linked arms. That voice made the daydreams so tasty and tangible.

Sharing my bed with love was a revelation. There were flushed faces and mortification if we bumped into our neighbour the next morning. The walls of those terraces were like paper and the poor man's bedroom was through the wall from ours. I could never look him in the eye. He could only have noisy-neighbour hate in his heart.

The Voice and the Daydreamer took Sunday long strolls

together and paused only to eat. When you're in love and gripped by good sex, food is never more wonderful. They liked to eat a lot. They wandered and embraced and wandered and ate all the best food in the land.

They ate and locked limbs and ate some more and made new daydreams together. They made up stories and planned amazing projects. He wanted to direct movies and she wanted to write books. That voice and those daydreams combined were a creative dream come true.

The right man in your bed is a glorious thing. The smell and taste of him, the wrapping and grappling of limbs. Even Simon's obsession with listening to the *Blade Runner* soundtrack every night before sleep was oddly glorious to begin with. Love was not blind, but for me it was clearly deaf.

Daydreams are lovely because you can take them in the right direction. You can choose where they go. Reality is never like that. Daydreams never really bite you in the ass, unless you have an ass-biting fetish and I don't. Reality is harder to steer altogether. I have often been daydreaming when reality takes a sharp turn.

I am standing on a flashy street corner in New York City chewing a giant pretzel and my boyfriend is acting strangely. I barely notice because New York is full of noise. We are here for a screening of Simon's short film at a festival and it occurs to me that Simon is a bit twitchy. He's nervous about his film,

I think. Then I take another pretzel bite. I dive back into some Yankee diner daydream that's flipping home fries.

I am too busy diner-dreaming to notice Simon buy two 'I Love New York' shot glasses right under my nose and a snipe of champagne. So when he drops to his knees at the top of the Empire State Building it's more than a shock. I just didn't see it coming. It hadn't entered my head.

The Voice from his knees is the squeakiest and most nervous I've ever heard him and the Daydreamer is puzzled. Marriage? It hadn't ever occurred to me. But now that it has a voice, suddenly it seems like the most fantastic, stupendous and best idea in the whole goddamn world and New York City. Say it in your normal voice, I squeak back, and the voice repeats it in regular CAPITAL LETTERS. Ruth Patricia O'Neill, will you marry me? YES! I shout – in capitals too – and from the top of this skyscraper, daydreams and reality embrace as though they are always one and the same thing.

My children are notorious bed-hoppers. They seem to wander through the night, their hot little bodies crawling for fresh crevices, burrowing in multiple beds. The more beds the better.

With each year of marriage we graduated to bigger and better beds. More sophisticated duvet covers. A solid ship on the shores of a shared life. Plenty of well-placed plump cushions and patterned throws.

We once lived in the Louth countryside. Three years married, our shared life came to a glorious crescendo with the mother of all ship-beds. A seven-foot behemoth, a magical beast of dark wood and miles of mattress. We had hundreds of cushions and could fit in the entire family of four. A frantic wriggler and a still little sloth both slotted in perfectly. Some children are wriggly and their chubby toes scratch your back all night. Others are solid hot water-bottles who never stir once they find their spot. We had both kinds.

That seven-foot bed was soaked by sunlight coming through our glass patio doors. They looked out on a country paradise of round green fields for miles. Despite the moving toddler traffic, I always slept peacefully and well. In the midst of wakeful baby nights, I could soothe myself back to dreamy sleep. I could cuddle some milky toddler skin, or roll them right out of the way to find man skin and long limbs and a neck you could sink your face into and then breathe deep.

Still living in the countryside and third time pregnant, I'm waiting for Simon in a neurologist's office. This green top makes my belly look like a glorious round hill on the Louth–Monaghan border. In my head I am drawing a childish picture of drum-lins beneath a cartoon sun. My dad has parked the car and joins me in the waiting room. Ooh, the grassy hill has just met a whole load of mud, I think gleefully as his muddy feet leave great streaks all over the floor. He is mortified but I can't stop giggling.

Afterwards, it will be the first time I ever regret a daydream. Why didn't I take more notice? Why wasn't I more prepared for the hit? I'm imagining shapes in Dad's footprints when the neurologist calls me in. Simon is standing up, with the palest face. Sound sucks out of my ears when the consultant speaks from behind his desk. 'Sorry, it's not good news.' Simon's voice is no longer in capital letters What's the prognosis? I ask with a whimper. Three to four years to live is the reply. TO LIVE? screams my brain in capital letters. MND is not an acceptable reason to break a daydream and it also wants to break a life.

The mother of all beds could fit the family fine until an unwelcome bedfellow came along. MND was a sneaky sort of a guest. At first all it wanted was a few extra pillows. Plump cushions had more function now than just being pretty props. Then MND wanted a sliding board so Simon could get into bed at all. We had banana-shaped ones and bendy ones but the best was a simple plain plank of wood that I would wedge under him like a seesaw and slide him down with one fell swoop. My arms got some shape to them. The bed was less roomy but we were all still aboard.

Sunlight still lit up our mornings but all the manoeuvring messed with the magic just a tiny bit. MND was tired and cranky. Our marital bed was under siege. It was a place where we now cried a lot.

For the first time it felt like daydreams couldn't save me

and nobody seemed to notice. We were all too busy. MND had turned our big bed into a battleship. Well, if this is war, I thought, then hear me roar. Bring it on, you bastard. I want my daydreams and my bed back.

Kisses

Alone at my cove, I blow sweet kisses out to sea. Thank you, sea. I can make sense of things here. The rolling rhythm of waves. How fantastic that the waves and I are hopelessly romantic. They somehow steady me. I am steady on the cove steps, gazing proudly back to shore.

A man on the beach is strolling with his son. He throws his boy high on his shoulders and his son laughs into the wind. It carries across the water and hits me hard. I am startled. The casual sweep of this man's arms, the wild abandon of his son's laughter, some of it, or all of it, startles me. It's a hollow sick feeling. Unsteady.

The gait of this man. His body harnessed in confident motion . . . My husband can only move his eyes. I kiss the soft cheeks of my children and his unfurrowed, troubled brow. Incessant waves become staggering. I stop blowing kisses out to sea.

*

In the wilds of Donegal, back when I was at a summer Irish school, I walked into the woods with a boy from the North wearing a bomber jacket. He was tall and much older than me and an experienced kisser. The kissing went on for hours and it was only that, just kissing. But I was just twelve years old and it felt too much. I wandered back to the *Bean an tí's* house in a daze to my bunk bed and straw mattress. My entire stomach had evaporated and the numb feeling crawled up into my throat. I couldn't even eat toast. I want to stay with the memory of this twelve-year-old girl, but my thoughts move to murkier waters. I remember a man called Dave the DJ.

Dave lived in a granny flat with his Peruvian wife. She had a rice cooker of which he was very proud. His wife cooked the perfect rice, Dave would boast. The language barrier possibly diluted his general intensity, so his wife considered Dave to be quite normal. She was a stern-looking woman, but then living with a man who drank only Coca-Cola and had a fine burger sheen to his skin might make you grumpy.

Get out of my head, Dave, I don't want you here. I worked in radio for five years but that was eleven years ago. I'd rather be brave and think of my husband's lost kisses. Lips that lock into each other. A wrapping, twisting, hungry kiss. The only other food Dave ate besides burgers and his wife's perfect rice, were spring rolls. These rolls were made with care and deep-fried by the tiny, delicate hand of a Filipino half his age. She sometimes visited the radio studio. All Dave talked about was her spring rolls. They were so tasty he couldn't stop himself once he started a plateful, he said. She would giggle a lot with her milky-coffee skin and a smile like sunshine. Dave didn't care much for real sunshine. He worked a lot of DJ nights and preferred artificial light. First thing in the morning before going on air, he would pull down all the shades in the studio, make it cave-dark, rub his hands together and say let's get some burgers.

I used to lock lips with my husband. Now those lips hang loose. His eyes burn bright. 'Kiss me on the lips' demands the computer voice, 'My mother kisses me on the forehead.'

Have I forgotten how to kiss? Does the body remember? It remembers in dreams, all right. In dreams I am master of the movie kiss, swelling music and softly merging silhouettes.

Dave would constantly fret about his Filipino fan's admiration. What am I going to do? he would ask me, head in his hands. Stop eating spring rolls, I would say. Go home to your wife, Dave, and remember how much you love her rice. Nothing ever came of it but he was addicted to all the drama.

Does my husband dream of lost kisses? Lost kisses with me? I doubt they are with me. Dream kisses work best if they don't pull you back to your partner, in sickness or in health.

Dave's other great obsession was conspiracy theories. Give me stuff on UFOs he would say and growl sightings of crackpot alien stories into the mic with more conviction than a newscaster breaking the latest bomb threat.

I will kiss my husband's loose lips if he wants me to, but my lips find the man at his brow. I crave the curve of his forehead not to be motherly, but to remind me of this man. He's still here and there's fire in those eyes.

The last time I saw Dave was my last day in radio. When he heard I was leaving, he walked up to me and kissed me as hard as he could right on the mouth. He walked away without a word. A startled, unwanted kiss. Unsteady. I never spoke to him again. A selfish man. I miss him sometimes. Dark devious desire that repels and attracts.

Go away, Dave. I remember raw passion as something more beautiful. Lunging, tearaway kisses in a toilet cubicle. That first lock-lipped kiss in a night club. Sweaty kisses in a beach hut in Thailand. I gaze out to sea. These memories disperse on foam and surf. I want to grasp them. Instead, I am stuck with Dave.

My twelve-year-old self was wise. She knew when dark desire was too much. She didn't go back for more kisses in the woods. She fell back on dreams. Her appetite returned. Steady. Such a lovely thing, a movie kiss. Sitting on the cove steps, I try and banish Dave. But there's no policing him here. Not at my cove with the relentless roll of waves.

I am rolling in thoughts of the past. I roll under with the fear that my own longing will turn grim and stale and devious. The empty feeling will grow. It will veer from the movie kiss to selfish places. Soft waves still roll to shore. The sea is calm today but the wind is high and I wish that the man and his laughing son would just leave the beach and that Dave would get out of my head.

My son Raife crept into bed one morning and folded himself against me in half sleep. 'I had a lovely dream,' he said. 'A girl called Tiger with golden hair. She kissed me but I woke up and she was gone. I felt sad.' My longing is not selfish. Not like Dave. It is still pure as my son's heart and a twelve-year-old girl unable to eat toast with the *Bean an tí*.

The deep longing that gets buried in daily tasks. The dark longing of the soul to make contact. Steady, then unsteady. The rolling of waves. But it's pure, not devious. Not even graphic or naked or hardcore. It's as simple as a kiss. I look to the beach again at the man and his son. Waves return to a steady rhythm. I blow another kiss back to shore.

Happiness

Home is a patterned plastic tablecloth. I see a young wife at her new kitchen table. Her soul sits and ponders happiness in the morning sun. Happiness casts slanting light on the plastic orange print. She is practising her new signature with a self-conscious flourish on a piece of paper. She writes it over and over again. Ruth Fitzmaurice, Ruth Fitzmaurice.

'Husband. Husband. Why do you keep calling me husband?' her new husband laughs. The young wife doesn't know. Maybe she feels like part of a team. Like they both know the joke and nobody else does. They both know something they call the deep magic.

The woman at the table thinks her new husband is all of her best thoughts and feelings. She has crept out of bed to sit alone in the early sun, surrounded by shared lovely things. Glassware and wedding delft rattle softly in the cabinet as a train goes by. She is pleasantly surprised to like it here, and to like the feeling of her marital home. She used to be a girl not fond of things, too busy floating on the wind, hungry for the hunt, chase, adventure. In short, she was mostly miserable. They call this love the deep magic.

I am surrounded by the same lovely things as the young wife. Home is still a plastic tablecloth. In this house, the pattern has changed to Cowboys and Indians. The unused cabinet of glass has clouded in ten years. I have pondered the perfect harmony of lining those glasses up on the back wall with steely calm. I could frisbee a few fancy plates at them. I could stick long-stemmed glasses into the ground like delicately upturned flowers glinting in the sun just to stomp on them. There is a magic deeper still.

The young wife has unravelled herself from the warm furry limbs of her new husband. The perfect look of sleepy abandon on his face is somehow ageless. She loves him like this, but sits at the table to think of him further. She has never felt closer to another human being.

I have an artist friend who was widowed in her twenties. She brought her grief to a young widows' club only to find out she was the youngest member there. Kind ladies grabbed and pulled her into their circle. They wore their pain on pendants and preserved it in old photographs.

I have sliced married life in two parts with a knife: before and after MND. I can hold myself in the present at my table.

I can hold photographs in my hands. But how can I be sure these memories are not a preserved pendant around my neck?

I can remember the first moment her shy, independent spirit crashed into something that was deep magic. It was all handsome eyes and dark brow. It wasn't even a body, it was a stance. Tactile limbs and dancing hands. Shirt and ripped jeans hung from a frame with swagger. Within the frame was a beautiful mind with principles, dreams, love, confidence but mostly, yeah, she thinks, it was the swagger. This something was a man who made the young woman blush.

The man saw himself as the Joker in the pack. Certain in his uncertainty, but never indifferent. The Joker is the philosopher, said the man. He's on a relentless quest for truth. The woman didn't know much about philosophy or universal truth. The man to her looked more like a Jack of Spades. All talk and charm and cheeky mischief, a bit of a chancer and yet full of natural wonder. As for her? The man jokingly called her the Nun. She was a full set of Hearts.

The man tried to impress her with stories. She knew he'd told them all before and she told him so. The man was impressed, and the woman thought this was funny. She didn't need his stories she could see his soul so clearly. She would have dived into those eyes like swimming pools and did not care that this sounded cheesy.

The man wrote her poems and took her to dinner. This is

the Joker finally getting the Nun, he wrote. Yes, after all these years, he finally gets her when no one is looking. The Nun blushed and thought this love is holy and if this is religion good God sign me up now. She was so overcome that she dropped her fork at dinner.

How can I trust these memories? I know the Nun existed because I found her in the attic. She was Sellotaped up in a box. Her thoughts popped out of an old journal along with her casual insecurities, nibbling of nails, worries about work, being newly married, having babies. She is there all along, under dust, holding on to the Joker as he used to be. Her happiness was real – it was perfectly imperfect.

Thanks to my journal, I see him now. Simon the reader, writer, poet, aspiring film-maker, weaver of dreams. He's sitting at our tablecloth, licking his finger and turning the squeaking, glossy pages of a large cinema book. He's hunched over his little desk, clean-shaven and shirted before work, manically tapping his laptop. He's made me Ready-brek with honey for breakfast. A watch rattles on his wrist.

Seven-year-old Arden gets distracted. He never gets dressed in time for school. 'It's not my fault!' he wails and points at his two older brothers. 'They distracted me!' I used to get mad until their uncle explained it to me. Arden doesn't see himself when he's with them, he explains. He has no sense of self yet.

He is living vicariously through them. Just like the Nun, his glassy eyes crave distraction. A spell has been cast. This is the deep magic.

The Joker was purer than the Nun – ironically – and she loved him for it. Why would I watch a horror film about forests? he would shrug. I love forests. Why ruin that? He was so pure he was afraid of bad thoughts. The Nun had a funny bone that was cracked black and charcoaled and she told the Joker that bad thoughts could be fun. They could set you free. Never be afraid of your imagination, she said.

The Joker showed the Nun real goodness and she stole his fear of the bad. And that was all the man needed for his imagination to take full flight. He had big dreams and together they would fly. The girl had dreams too but liked being distracted. True love was the deep magic. His dreams were big enough for two and the future was plenty long enough for her dreams too.

Today I sit at my plastic tablecloth knowing the future no longer exists. Would my younger self have been better off knowing this future? Would I want to break the happy spell at her table? The cruelty of this life might crush her and big waves are coming. Surrounded by lovely things, she would laugh in my face. Get out of my home, mad woman! Don't you know the power of deep magic? Don't you know the rules? Nothing bad befalls the likes of us!

The young wife thinks her life is as magical as it can be.

Look at the glory of him. Her own self got sidetracked during this long fixed gaze. And who could blame her? Not me. This spell alone won't carry her through the harsh waves ahead. It's not enough. She will have to dive much deeper than that.

At the young widows' club, the dead are deities to be worshipped. My artist friend, the young widow, was horrified. She respected their coping skills but just couldn't cope with them. Her husband had died but she was still alive. So she carried her grief out of the circle. Her late husband sat on her shoulders. She wore her pain proudly and booked a round-trip to see the world.

The young wife at her kitchen table knows about deep magic. But I know her future. Life is going to push and pull her like a wave. She doesn't have a choice and neither do I. Come with me, dear girl, sit at my tablecloth. The journey is upon us and to survive it, you can't just ride the wave, you have to become one. Can we do this? Let's go. Becoming a wave just might be the deepest magic of them all.

Colour

Nurses, nurses everywhere. Nurses filling kettles in the kitchen. Nurses scuffling with coffee cups. Ringed cups scattered about like a student flat. The bathroom door is locked and there's a queue. Who's in there? It's a nurse. Nurses at the microwave nuking fragrant food during our dinner. Nurses at the sink spilling suds. Nurses standing over our bed at night as we sleep. Nurses catching me in my knickers. Lock the door. Nurses are everywhere. They're just doing their job. Pain is chasing me through busy stressful rooms. Nurses are in every corner of our tiny home.

What is a home? What exactly does home mean? I need an answer. The only answers forthcoming could fit on a few Post-its. They are all worthy slogans. They would make great fridge magnets:

Home is not a house.

Home is a feeling.

Home is the people you love.

Home is where the heart is.

A house is made of bricks and beams, a home is made of love and dreams.

That last one is an actual fridge magnet.

When Simon came home on a ventilator, the hospital nurses all cried. 'God doesn't give you more than you're able for,' said one nurse to me as we hugged goodbye. God is pretty creative, I think, or else he just saw me as a challenge.

Nurses and carers are everywhere. They are a merry band of the kindest souls mixed with some wonderful freaks. Our home is a revolving door for a whole spectrum of psyches. A nurse slips me presents of holy medals while whispering, hand on heart, that the Devil talks to her in person. The Devil tells her to do bad things. A night nurse with a ghoulish white face hides behind hall corners and jumps out at me each time I pass. I must shout every word in defiance of her deaf ears and it is her job to listen through a baby monitor to make sure Simon stays alive. WHAT? This is the night of the living dead.

Home for me has always been colour. Home is a warm colour. It's a swirly orange-yellow colour like sunshine. I'm sitting with a cup of hot tea in my hands listening to birdsong in chorus. The dawn light is so bright it lights up the kitchen wall pure orange.

I never knew that hippies were such control freaks. Beware the nurses brandishing big jewellery and natural remedies. Theirs is a will not to be battled with. If you don't do it their way, they walk. Simon is a young man trapped in a body that doesn't move. The hippies are up against pure fire. So they walk.

Looking for peace, I need to lock pain away. Pain refuses to stay padlocked, so I park it outside of small moments. These moments are mostly rituals surrounding coffee. I make my coffee in a little pot and carry it in a cup away from madness. I must contemplate a weekend of two new nurses. Two more new nurses will be coming to our house. I will settle into the edges of our home. For a small moment, I will simply gaze out the window at my birch tree, at least until this cup is drained.

Nurses with noisy shoes. Giant man nurses who don't fit. They have to stoop in doorways. Tiny women nurses who can't reach the cup press. The agency send a Spanish carer with spina bifida who can barely walk. She cries because she can't climb up on our double bed and help to hoist Simon. The nurse sends her away still crying. They're very emotional people, she says.

Pain chases me around the house like a big angry scribble. I make lists to unscramble it. I move my body away from it. My list says things like, buy a second microwave and a kettle to put in the nurses' office. That might help. Organising order might help, but you cannot organise chaos. So I just keep moving.

A nurse in clog shoes and a plain skirt explains that she rejects all forms of technology. For religious reasons. 'I don't need a radio because I sing and talk to the birds!' she chirps. Mottled plastic bags and coat hangers full of clothes fill her car. There was a fire, she laments. She fishes out her wedding photo from a plastic bag to show me. Her wedding dress is the colour and texture of crumbly brown bread. I wonder if the dress is in her car too. She sings and keeps giving me presents of rose-scented soap. She chases my mother around the kitchen trying to give her a shoulder massage, shouting, 'You look tense!' Now it's my mother's turn to run the other away.

I move and I get busy doing things. A good friend gave me a coffee cup with a great slogan. It says, 'A clean house is the sign of a wasted life'. There is enough waste around here so I don't do that. Instead, I paint colours. I sand down our postbox and paint it pillar box red. I sand and paint the garden bench and back door the same bright beacon red. I get on hands and knees outside and surround our red-brick house with a turquoise-green plinth. I get giddy in the back garden with greens and bright blues. Home is colour. It just makes me feel better.

Many nurses bring gifts, from holy medals, to peppercorns and bathrobes for the kids. Unlike my mother I say yes to the offers of massage, especially during pregnancy when my feet are swollen and sore. A nurse gives me a head massage using masses of Deep Heat cream and it blows my head off. After that, I question my mantra of saying yes to things.

I paint stuff and cook spicy food. Sometimes I bake but I'm a terrible baker. It requires precision and so my biscuits fall apart. Cooking calms me and makes the house smell more like family. A carer runs out of the room red-faced and eyes bulging – it turns out she is highly allergic to chilli. The fumes alone are chasing her down the road. She could blow up like a balloon and need adrenaline shots for anaphylactic shock. My cooking might actually kill her. In the face of potential death, I shamefully get the giggles.

My kitchen fridge is a messy tapestry of colour. Kids' pictures, scribbled poems, magnets and old photos cover it in muddled chaos. I don't have any fridge magnet slogans except for one. Slapped right in the middle my magnet reads, This Too Shall Pass.

Good nurses come and go. Cait has a voice that rings like a bell and fills the house with violin music. A Honda Shadow parked outside means young Adam with his Peter Pan heart has arrived. Paula brings mischief and laughter. The twins let Anna wipe their bums after going to the toilet. This is high praise indeed. Gentle Benedict shares so many Tuc crackers with the kids they are renamed Benedict crackers. Good nurses come and then they go.

*

Moving is running, but you can't run away for ever. Running away never solved anything. Did it? I need to take moments away from nurses. Get through it. No expectations but to survive. This Too Shall Pass.

School runs make me run, run, run. I wish I could pause in the space between school pickups. Slip into a crack in the warmth of a parked car and stop time. Running is moving. Don't stop moving. Running away is about taking moments. A super six-pack of Jack, Raife, Arden, Sadie, Hunter and I can run, but the seven of us can't. I am all too aware that it's escape without Simon. I struggle with it, but I need it. We would run for ever if only Simon could run with us. But he can't. So that is why we invent Runaway Days.

Then Marian arrives. She is very quiet at first but has smiling eyes. She talks when spoken to, laughs and knits neck warmers for all the children. They are five different colours. She is fascinated by all my cooking. 'I'm a terrible cook,' she chuckles, 'but I can give a hell of a bed bath.' It's important to know your strengths, I reply and we both laugh. Marian is a woman who knows what she is good at.

How do you run solo with five children under ten? Is it safe? We run with chaos. We go to Tesco and faces drop. Heads turn in our wake. My children are lying in the aisles and thrashing each other in the trolley. Chaos can be fun. We play the shop game. Each child gets to choose one thing and we return home laden with giant jammy rolls and cupcakes. We run through Ikea and blatantly follow the arrows the wrong way. We race to the cove to climb rocks and hurl stones and howl into the wild salty air. The sound of the sea is the only thing that can drown out this lot.

On Runaway Days we are mayhem. We are lords and rulers of the playground. Don't mess with us. After we visit people they gasp in the silent aftershock, once our noisy goodbyes leave. But mostly it's just us six. Chaos is pure colour. We walk through forests with sticks that make swishing sounds. We drive to Dealz discount shop to buy plastic swords and giant cartons of teabags. We hit the Asian superstore, full of spices and weird plastic-looking sweets. It makes the shop game way more interesting.

Runaway Days are allowed because we have other days with Simon. We always come home. We bring back colour until it's time to run again. I don't know if I can live like this. I don't know who I am or what I am good at or how to make a home here. Is Simon OK? Are the kids OK? What is this doing to us all?

Marian is the kindest person I have ever met and she is everywhere. Her knitting is on the couch. Her half-eaten ready-meals litter the kitchen and I couldn't give a shit. It doesn't matter because I don't need to run away from Marian. Not ever.

Marian sees colours and energies. She comes to work one day and laughs out loud. 'Look at what you did with your painting, Ruth!' she says with childish excitement. 'You surrounded your house with the colours red and green and blue. Red and green are the angel colours of love and healing. Blue is protection. You've made a force field!' Through her eyes I see it. I have done my best to make us a new home here. Best of all, I might even be getting good at it.

Aifric

My friend Aifric is like a wishing well. I've been throwing wishes her way since we were three years old. From a family of seven and with four sisters, Aifric has been surrounded by chaos her whole life. She is the calmest person I know. All five sisters have an ethereal quality to them. A light magical step not quite of this world.

Seven-year-old Arden marches into the kitchen and announces he's leaving home. 'Sorry, Momma,' he commiserates, hand on my shoulder. 'My friend Jack Diamond's house is WAY cooler. I just like it there more.' I smile and give him a hug, because I know. As a child, that's exactly how I felt about Aifric's house. Arden goes further and actually packs a bag. 'Don't worry, I still love you,' he adds as an afterthought. Armed with a stick and a Samurai sword, he heads off down the road.

Just married, we lived in Greystones where Simon had

grown up. The sea was breathtaking but I was driving past it rather than jumping in. I was so busy having babies that our house got too small. We needed a bigger boat. Making a tribe of kids is one thing. For Simon and me this happened fast. But how do you find your tribe? How do you find your people and figure out where you belong? For us this happened slowly. We struggled to search for a place to take root.

My favourite place to be as a kid was the kitchen at Aifric's house. It was big enough to take in everyone. It was warm enough to take in anyone. A full stove of heat and the smell of warm peat. At teatime they would empty the fridge on to the counter. Whoever was around got to choose whatever they wanted to eat. Seven children, a few friends and maybe a random bronzed hitchhiker her mother had salvaged from the main road. Hitchhikers always got a bed for the night. Aifric's kitchen had the capacity to absorb anything. We could make any kind of sandwich we liked. We rolled slices of bread around whole bananas. I loaded some cream cheese and honey on top. Why not?

Simon grew up by the sea and wanted to stay by the sea. We searched for a house there first. So many shores to choose from on this island. Our search spanned Sligo to the vast golden sands of Donegal. We whispered on wild rugged coastlines about a different life in a cottage somewhere. The kids could run free. They'd have an amazing childhood until puberty hit. Then they could spend days mowing our massive lawn wearing large resentful headphones. They could have real hate in their hearts. It was a romantic vision.

A property boom had boosted our first family home in Greystones through the stratosphere. We sold it for crazy money. We were giddy with the notion of living mortgage free in a creative wonderland. Brimming with love and promise, we set forth across the land. We would settle for nothing less than pure magic. Possibilities are endless when you feel invincible.

Sometimes I have a temper. I bang a pot off the kitchen sink so loud that all my children cry. Jack dashes from the room. I try my best but sometimes I lay my stresses out like broken glass at their feet. My friend Aifric never rages. She ponders and contemplates. One morning her three girls were screaming so much, she slowly spread peanut butter on her toast and climbed up on the kitchen counter. She just crouched up there quietly and nibbled her toast until it was eaten.

Aifric is like a wishing well because you could tell her anything. It wouldn't even occur to her to pass it on. She doesn't just keep secrets, they fall for ever somewhere deep. She moves gently and gracefully. She remains calm and wise as, all about her, the world rages. It's a source of great irony to me that she is surrounded by three fiery pixie daughters.

They dance around her in circles. Sometimes she looks slightly perplexed. She is their smooth centre.

We found our first house in an unlikely place. Half an hour from where I grew up. There was no sea in sight. Leaving the sea was one of the biggest acts of love Simon ever showed me. I see it in retrospect only because I could never leave the sea now. Not even for him. In Co. Louth on the edges of Monaghan, we named this house North Cottage. It had rolling hills and apple trees. The kitchen had a range cooker and a half-door out the back. Out front was practically picket-fenced. At dusk on a nearby hill, a dray horse stood in silhouette. For two romantics this was a dream come true.

We knew nobody at first but didn't need anybody. Friends were secondary. We were our own tribe. We existed in perfect harmony. Our children ran with the wind and had grass-stained knees. Our cat went wild, leaving mouse gut massacres at the back door. Simon was writing his first movie script. I was pretending to write a book but mostly mooning over my babies. We had cots, old bookshelves and a warm stove. We walked the fields in our wellies.

I believe a few things about friendship. Good ones are based on mutual attraction. They are born from love. If I were gay I would totally fancy Aifric. She is a righteously gorgeous babe. Her attractiveness is more than physical, it's mystical.

She reminds me I should never have the arrogance to think I know people inside out. As her friend, my whole life I've been reading the most beautiful mystery novel that can never ever be solved. This mystery is no trickery. The wishing well just runs deep.

When you're young, girls can be scary. They say one thing and mean another. It's just mean. What do they mean? It's the greatest mind-melt brutal Mensa puzzle of all time. I have stifled memories of being trapped in a hot sweaty sleeping bag full of sobs and snot. At a girls' sleepover party, I hide in my hurt cocoon as the other girls laugh and jump over me. I can't remember why except that they're mean.

I grew up with four brothers. Boys are easy, straightforward. If it's mean, it's clearly meant to be. When they're hungry they eat. One best boy memory is wrestling my brother's friend to the ground in our garden when he teased me. Then we shake hands. Easy. Girl wrestling was monumentally more tricky.

MND ruined the romantic vision. It made North Cottage a prison. Illness does funny things to friendship. You feel small. How do you attract friends when you find yourselves unattractive? Having just each other was suddenly not enough. This thing was too big to bear.

Family helped but we both craved friendship. How could we find new friends now? How do you keep friends with illness glaring in the half-door? Forging new friendships felt impossible. There were no roots here. Did we belong anywhere? We would continue to wander like ghosts with no grasp on real matter. Our shape kept changing and people walked right through us.

Before I found the sea and my swimming tribe I had Aifric. I am always content to share the same space and admire the mystery of her. How do you find something like where to belong? MND had robbed us of free choice. We moved back to Greystones where it was safe. A network of family and friends existed to knit themselves around us.

Aifric and her husband lived in Greystones too and, in beautiful symmetry, we found that we were not-so-far-away neighbours. We gathered in my kitchen with our collective gaggle of kids and made dinner. It was a shared space beyond words.

Aifric is a friend I never had to find. Beyond Aifric, I worried if I belonged in Greystones. How could I begin to find out? Most things you don't have to find because they are there all along. Throw another wish out there any way you can. Will it make a splash? Just wait and see what you fall into.

Ergonomics

Simon has a system of shirts. His shirts are so fancy they have secret buttons. They come wrapped in soft tissue and smooth boxes. They arrive in firm glossy carrier bags. Swanky bags are embossed with big names, ribbon ties and rope handles. The shirts make Simon feel good. They are gifts from his mother. They make him feel so good that his mother keeps on buying them.

Some shirts are funky. Some are flowery. Some are zany with pictures of bicycles or stars or tiny teapots. So many are stripy, or spotted or checked. All of them are lovingly and expertly ironed by his mother's skilled hand. She places them symmetrically in our bedroom chest of drawers.

Statistics are a belief system in which many people hold faith. The statistics for MND don't jangle many faith bells. They just make you feel really, really unlucky. In Ireland approximately 110 people die of MND every year. In the US, somebody dies every 90 minutes; in the UK six people die each day, just under 2,200 per year; 100,000 people will die worldwide in the next 12 months. Cap it all in a considered margin of three or four years left to live. One neurologist tells us that a diagnosis of MND is like winning the lottery backwards. That's going too far for me. I measure out his words carefully. 'What a dick' is statistically my most likely response.

Illness by its nature is disorderly. A public system swoops in to serve and take good care. Doesn't it? Occupational therapists, social workers, dieticians, physios, public health nurses a butcher, baker, candlestick maker. They are all super nice and speak in loud voices. Meetings are very important to them. Many meetings take place, where plans are made. Plans must be written down. It's called a Care Plan. I may sound bitter but mostly I feel bemused. 'I'm just ticking boxes, Ruth,' is my favourite meeting catchphrase of all time.

Sometimes systems are nice. We cope in the world as creatures of habit. I make my coffee every day in the same order. The wrong cup ruins my mood. My son will not get dressed unless he puts his socks on first. Is that sweet? Before MND Simon would leap from our bed every morning and pull back the curtains. On his knees, his arms outstretched, he would salute the sun, or lack of it, eyes closed, whispering a silent prayer. His was a simple system of thanks.

Safety systems soothe our sick souls. A religion for the unwell. Systems will save us and bring forth serenity. Time is a prison of planned habits. Cherish order in all things. When does it become obsessive? Freaky? Cultivate your compulsive side. Disregard any disorder. Embrace your inner freak. Perhaps we're all a bit sick.

The public system can't work fast enough. MND can always work faster. Theirs is a system with its very own language. Language is important, just like ticking boxes. Great care must be taken, even with what name to call Simon. An Invalid is not valid. There's no patience for Patients. How's your form? Just fill in this form. Incurable implies imperfect and Disease equals disgust. We shall call Simon the Service User. Is he confined to a wheelchair? Perfect. Box ticked. We'll call him the Client. The word Client sits well in the realms of confinement.

We'll just pop out to the house to do an assessment. Assess what? Who is being assessed? Them or us or me or him? Our children? The word assessment sets me on edge. Social workers send me edgier still. Are they judging me? Should I say thank you? Why are they here? Will I offer them a cup of tea? What do you need? they say. We'll write it down. Someone to talk to? Well, they're not offering that. No counselling for me beyond talking to trees. Best not to mention the trees.

Factor in the ventilator a few years later and MND leaves statistics behind. On the vent, Simon invents a safety system all his own. Who could blame him? He cannot move or eat or breathe. He can feel everything, including fear. In the face of fear how do you feel in control? When trust is in the hands of another and nurses are just passing through, how can you feel safe? His own system helps. The most marvellous, magnificent, mind-blowing system of all time. Tasks must be performed specifically in a set order. Do not dictate to the man in the bed. Good nurses can learn the system. Simple. Forget the order and you start again. Those nurses can leave.

Way back, when Simon has been in the wheelchair a few months, I am sent on a manual handling course. I am an eager student. I've learned a few manoeuvres already. Proud of the tricks up my sleeve and how we've adapted, I am keen to show off my moves. I make some rude 'man handling' jokes to my husband as I set out from North Cottage to the training centre in Co. Louth.

It's a course for carers and nurses and for me. I sit with happy Howaya's and comfy Nigerian women who clasp their hands under their bosoms and laugh along. My hand is constantly in the air with questions. Each of my moves is met with a frown and a big fat fail. All approved moves of the Client require a minimum of two people. At home it's just me. I am an army of one. I try not to cry every time the jolly instructor talks about the Service User and ergonomics. What the fuck is ergonomics? I will have to go home and look it up.

The perma-tanned girl behind me whispers that it's hard not to get attached when you're in the home. Oh God. She thinks I'm a nurse like her. She doesn't realise I am the home she's talking about. I need to go to that home now. The Service User, the Client, belts, slide sheets, banana boards. I buy a packet of cigarettes and sit in my car smoking half a Marlboro Light, with sunglasses on. I don't even smoke, or wear sunglasses. The glasses steam up from crying. These fags are gross. Nothing works. Maybe I need hard drugs. There's a permanent knot in my stomach.

Ergonomics is human engineering. I looked it up. *'The scientific discipline concerned with the understanding of interactions among humans and other elements of a system and the profession that applies theory, principles, data and methods to design in order to optimize human well being and overall system performance,'* says the internet. Maybe I need another cigarette. It's hard to find any magic in ergonomics.

My son Raife runs into the kitchen at 6 a.m. with an excited screech.

'I did it, I DID IT! I finally DID IT.'

'Did what?' we all respond as eagerly as you can at 6 a.m.

'Last night, while I was asleep, I got control of my dream.'

'Wow,' says Jack. 'That's impossible.'

Impossible? Raife could be the Power Ranger of all sleep, the Overlord of lucid dreamland. His reign as High King of dreams is not impossible. It's a lot more likely than me ever getting to grips with motherfucking ergonomics.

The shirt system keeps coming. MND took away all my

treats, Simon says. All I have is coffee, whiskey and my shirts. I don't begrudge him a treat. How could I? There are so many shirts I buy a second wardrobe for the twins' bedroom. I move most of my clothes in there to make room for more shirts. His mother can't stop buying shirts. How could she? They help him. The shirts clearly help her too. She widens her scope to well-cut jackets, pyjamas, plush cords and trousers that fit just right.

A big cartoon moon sits over Greystones seafront one night. A big cartoon grin spreads over my face as we stop the car. I'm used to staring out to sea in broad daylight. By night we hear dark waves crashing. This crazy bright beast fills the sky. A mile of moonpath is dancing over dark waters. I fish out my phone to take a photo. That's why I love the moon. You can't catch it on a smartphone. On my phone this monster looks the size of a pencil torch. Clever moon.

You can't catch MND with ergonomics. Soon after the manual handling course in Co. Louth I am running back and forth between babies in the house. Simon is in his separate studio across the garden. I skid over gravel bringing him tea and fall down some concrete steps. It's a bad fall. There is nobody to pick me up, so I just lie there. I chuckle at the state of myself. Social workers, come see me now. Ergonomics and systems won't ever win. They'll just grind your face into the gravel over and over again.

Meanwhile the moon and MND keep on dancing.

Tragic Wives

My friend Michelle is a warrior. Not just in spirit. I think she is an actual warrior; she may have chain mail under her T-shirt. I'm sure there's some manner of sword tucked under her pillow.

I first met Michelle in my boyfriend's kitchen. She was cooking up a vegan feast in his house. Mouth-watering smells seemed to charge from her fingertips. She could cook for forty people with no more than an old pot and a stick. This tiny dynamo was the dark pretty girlfriend of Simon's housemate Galen. It was just the four of us for dinner instead of forty, so we ate well.

Back then, Simon was a waiter. He was spinning plates and stories while studying for a master's in film. I was working in radio and Galen was the rare beast who lived downstairs, a journalist skipping between social events. He would turn up at all hours, his shirt unbuttoned and tie askew. We gathered regularly to eat mounds of Michelle's food and laugh as much as possible.

Michelle is like a cool breeze over solid rock. Whisper her name across the waves. She is Pocahontas-pretty with a wildness behind the eyes. This girl will giggle girlishly and then tell you she works as a forensic psychologist. She deals with so many of the country's hardcore murderers, criminals and rapists that at work she has a fake name. I imagine her in her job like a suited Clark Kent, all ponytail and black-rimmed spectacles. In work she's no warrior of the sea. She's a fine lady called Laura with sensible shoes.

'Momma, remember the time you dreamed Sadie fell down a pothole and you couldn't catch her because it was so deep and then she died?' I don't need to remember my own dreams because my son Raife does it for me. Why on earth did I tell him that about his little sister? Must have been some fine parenting moment. But also, how does he remember it in such detail?

'It's because I have a golden brain' is his reply.

Golden brains make for golden memories. Details are not as important to me as feelings, which is lucky, because I don't remember details. What year, which month, what time and how long? Who cares? Not me. Memories don't mind. I claim ownership as long as I can feel it, body and soul.

The world is big but often small people can walk tall.

With her well-seasoned past and a dash of daring, Michelle has swum oceans and climbed mountains. She has thrown street parties in New York. There were rock band road trips on tour buses and adventures in vineyards. No big deal. Michelle took it all in huge strides with those tiny legs.

There's a first time for everything. Have you ever felt so alive and inspired that it feels like sparks are coming out your fingertips? Your body is fully charged. You are pumped and fizzling. Your insides sizzle, your gizzard feels cooked and your hair follicles tingle. First times can be fearful or fun or a first-time fusion of both. We had sworn to take the plunge after Galen's marina swim. I don't recall the exact date of that first dip with Michelle and Aifric, but the feeling was positively golden.

Michelle loves dogs. She climbed down a sheer cliff in Greystones once to save a large lurcher stuck on the train tracks. He was carried to safety in her arms and the owner still sends her Christmas cards. She knew those cliffs well from truant school-days perched up there between classes. Like many people, Galen and Michelle took a gap year in Australia with their kids. Unlike many, they shipped a new car home along with a giant purebred white Swiss shepherd called Casper.

The first time I kissed Simon I got slammed up against a nightclub wall. We went home, stayed up all night with candles around us, talking, talking, more than talking, like there was so much to say we could never stop. His beard ravaged my face raw the next day into four pink points. My four-pointed star he called it. Better than a swim? Oh, well, yes, don't kid yourself. A swim is not better than this.

Michelle, Aifric and I huddle on the cove beach, trailing an ever-moving entourage of kids. Under-threes are running amok. Michelle's war baby Bodhi, sits Buddha-like at the epicentre, stuffed snug in his car seat. With a name like Bodhi he's a future surfer dude for sure. Or else an accountant. Either way he'll get some *Point Break* moments right here. Casper the dog is running hurricane circles around us, the most eager to swim of all.

Where were you when you found out? We all remember. Galen crashed his bike on the N11 dual carriageway. His head was down, he was pedalling fast. That head hit a parked truck on the hard shoulder so hard, his helmet split in two, along with his spine. Galen's crash is like our own Greystones JFK or Michael Jackson. Out of disbelief, we all swap stories.

There is a secret society of the hurt. We harbour pain skilfully under smiles. Observe a subtle strain behind the eyes. A certain tension in the jaw muscles. 'You grind your teeth in your sleep,' one night nurse tells me matter-of-factly. The hurt seek each other out wordlessly. We gather on a stony beach that may as well be a deserted car park. Expect some dodgy deals. We swap pain silently like illegal contraband.

Still fully dressed, we stand clustered against the wind. Shoes get removed first, collectively. It's our wordless signal to stop hesitating. This swim is on. Teeth hold my towel in place with a face grimace as I negotiate limbs into my flowery swimsuit. We may have walked in from the shore that first day and then swum to the steps. First-timers soon learn that diving straight in from the steps is best. My battered body gives a brief shy shiver, finding itself in a swimsuit in September, but it's short lived. We go out in pairs so there's always someone with the entourage. Michelle and Casper swim both times.

In the depths of winter, a rubber hat is our only concession to the cold. I like to freeze my feet walking on cold stones before the plunge. People pay money to walk over pebbles in fancy health spas. Hobbling over sharp rocks towards the steps, I can see why. Call me masochistic but this feels amazing. I will learn these pre-swim rituals but there is no getting used to this. I stand on those steps every time with raw fear. Your brain screams NO! It's the first time every time. To dive you need to turn your brain off. Shut up, brain. Steer past your brain because something else is steering you. What the fuck am I doing? This makes no sense. That's why it makes perfect sense. JUST DIVE.

Cold water hits you with a head-slam. Don't fight the cold. Let go and let it seep in. But it's so cold! Keep treading water. This too shall pass. Ten seconds later you don't feel the sting. Ten seconds later is pure freedom. Wind hits the sea surface and scatters salt spray on your face. Icy waves push and pull at bodies so relentlessly, they take your breath away. Seawater seeps into shocked mouths. They gag with a metallic salty aftertaste.

We climb out of the water back up the steps with numb, pink bodies. Hands grab the rusty railing to avoid a slip. Talking, talking, we just can't stop talking and laughing. We are kings of the world. Bonded by sea, we're laughing and sharing this feeling. Better than sex? Don't delude yourself, it's not better than all of it.

Why isn't everyone doing this? People stroll past on the footpath overhead. Down the path a few steps and you are drinking in rock and sea and salt and wild. Hey you with your dog and headphones! Switch off your brain! Join us! Dive in! We could happily become the worst kind of swimming evangelists. Let's change the world one dive at a time.

The shivering swimmers shine like diamonds. My lips have gone blue. Michelle's face looks wide open. She's walking taller. Aifric looks mostly astonished.

Dog-walkers greet Michelle by the shore. 'How's Galen?' they gasp with pity in their eyes and squeeze her salty sea arm. 'You're just *great*. You're *both* great. I don't know how you do it. You're so *brave*'.

'Jesus, Michelle,' I mutter, 'we're like the Tragic Wives' Club.'

'So what the hell is Aifric doing here?' says Michelle and we let rip a wild collective cackle.

*

Aifric has no business being in a Tragic Wives' Club. Her husband Phil is way too healthy. He grew up with Simon and Galen in Greystones. They are all best friends. Phil sits in their collective wheelchair company often. Both Simon and Galen are blessed with full heads of hair. 'At least we'll never be bald like Phil,' teases Simon one day. Bald as a tragedy just cracks them both up. It's wheelchair guy humour. Aifric has no business being here but that's OK. Neither do we. We can't claim ownership. Neither do we.

Superheroes

I have decided to become a superhero. I shout it out the half-door right into the starry sky. BRING IT ON, MND! I believe in love and love conquers all. I can be a superhero for love. The Nun hears her holy calling from way up high. But I'm not stupid. All superheroes need a decent costume.

It all started in Simon's foot. His right foot went floppy. I blamed his stiff clutch. The funky black convertible he drove way too fast with our eldest boy Jack in the back. It was an education in loud music. Go easy, Simon. This fast-moving dad made your heart skip beats. It was a pure thrill driving fast with Simon, his music pumping. Jack is as wide-eyed as me. His chubby hands dance along to tunes, with a headshake and glorious toddler cheeks wobbling.

When I hear the superhero call I quickly find my costume. I buy a novelty T-shirt online that says **I'm fine** in black letters across the front. Seeping from the ribcage is a disgusting fake mass of bright red blood. I love that T-shirt but it scares the children, so I don't wear it much. My regular housewife costume will do just fine. I'm a superhero in disguise.

The floppy foot wasn't the car, of course, it was MND saying hello. Simon is limping now and using a stick. I can hear him in North Cottage limping up and down the hall with a walker. He wants to get stronger, but MND has other ideas. Each scrape of that walker on the tiles pulls a little more romance out of our country home. Romantic dreams limp farther away.

'Poor Ruth, you're so *brave!*' people gush, until Aifric or someone who knows me well enough elbows them to silence. Don't pity her, they mutter with covered mouths. She hates that. For God's sake don't pity her. I want to tattoo that across my forehead. Don't pity me. Fuck off and don't pity *us*. I'm fine with blood seeping out of my ribcage. WE'LL BE JUST FINE.

Break-ups are always nasty. Romantic dreams are hard to break from. Simon limps into hospital with me when our third child, Arden, is born. It is six months since his diagnosis. He sits beside me to hold my hand. His face is the colour of ash and he's soon limping away again. His mind is locked into beating this thing his way. I'm sure the sight of his new son makes it stronger. He needs something to save him.

I'm skinny with secret muscles. I could lift grown men and children at the same time. Try and stop me.

Healers and holy men take his money as he limps around

the country with his mother. He got the cure for warts once by washing his hands in the dirty bird bath of some creepy old house when he was a kid. They believe in this stuff. They don't believe the medical doctors who deal in dismal diagnosis. They believe in wart cures. I believe in the power of what you believe in because it gives hope, so they have my blessing.

A healer called Nicholas tells Simon that everything is going to be OK. I cry when he tells me the story of this man who took his hand to give hope. Your poor wife, says the man simply. For some reason I take his pity. It hits my heart hard. We name our third son Arden Nicholas after this man who is the seventh son of a seventh son of a seventh son. He is born in December so everyone thinks it's a Santa thing, but we know differently.

Arden is our war baby and he has always been brave for it. In a windswept schoolyard, he is the kid standing with his coat wide open, his trousers possibly back to front and his tie askew. His mind is just above these material things. When he was three, he hurled himself down a massive water-slide in France. In primal parent fear, I hurled myself down after him. A manic mother scream rose out of me. I caught him in a catch pool and checked for signs of life. Are you OK? He was fine, with a smile and a shrug. My braveheart lion, I call him.

North Cottage is no longer home. Simon needs saving and this break-up is hard. At the heart of a break-up is an urge to go back to who you once were, an older version of yourself. It's someone you can understand and recognise. MND draws Simon back to his family. Their pursuit of an alternative diagnosis takes them through internet searches and blood tests for Lyme disease. When the holy men don't work they look for wart cures in tick bites and complementary medicine. It takes them to an industrial estate in England. This place calls itself a hospital. They suggest he has Lyme disease. They want him to go on intravenous antibiotics and vitamins and possibly have a back operation. Simon limps over to England with his mother and sister to live in an apartment. He gets a PIC line put in to flood his system with salvation.

Alternative diagnoses seek unconventional cures. It's a road that Simon is compelled to limp and trip upon. I am happy as long as he holds on to hope. The apartment is soulless so they rent a little cottage in the English countryside and bring Simon for treatments every day. In winter it is Christmas card pretty and snowing. We Skype at night, cottage to cottage in our back kitchens and talk about deep snow.

Simon is gone for months and I am knocking around North Cottage with our three boys. We run in the garden but we're not free. Where's Dadda? Jack whines. I light fires at night and feed the baby but there are no limping sounds from the hall. The countryside is silent. I don't feel scared under this starry sky. There are worse things to be scared of, but we still miss him so much. Everything is moving so fast but in the wrong direction. Simon's fast car is outside with a dead battery. I hop in my own car with the three boys and satnav my way across water. It's a long bridge from one cottage to another.

I arrive to find a country paradise. The snow has melted. Simon was whisked away to get fixed. Control is a crutch and a press full of vitamin jars. The limp is heavier now and he leans on a pair of crutches. Simon leans on his family. They make organic meals and healthy snacks. They have laminated lists of life-sustaining vitamins to be taken in specific order at breakfast, mid-morning, lunch and dinner. His mother is thrilled to give baby Arden his first bottle. It is so pretty and comfy here. I can see why Simon feels safe. To me it's as safe as a padded cell.

Now aged seven, Arden is reluctantly getting his hair cut in a fancy salon. He weaves his head away from the scissors as much as possible. Can you tidy it up? I ask the lady doubtfully. Arden's hair is pure pathetic fallacy. It's a wild emotional weather forecast. There is just no bringing this boy to heel. He likes to linger on the edge. Footpath edges, ten yards to the fringe of the group, that is where you will find Arden. Dangling on the edge of danger, he is a born heartbreaker. This boy will grow up, leave me, and travel the world without a backward glance. I can only hope he returns for the odd hot dinner.

The nice lady calls me over to look. See the way his hair grows, she demonstrates. I can't tidy it. It is growing in ten different directions. You just cannot tame this boy. Even his hair says so. I look at the back of Arden's hair growing up and down in swirly chaos and I feel inspired. My mind screams back to the memory of a polar opposite view. Rows and rows of vitamin jars.

I used to sneak into the room just to look at them. I would open the doors and gasp in wonder. That well-ordered press of vitamin jars. Face your fears. There couldn't have been fewer than fifty of them. Those clinical white smooth tubs of varying size. Each label faced forward the same way. I would touch them and fiddle with them and then fearfully straighten my fiddling. I had stared for too long and seen too much. The horror. That vitamin press scared the living shit out of me.

It was then I decided to become a superhero. If this is the superhero Simon needs, then I can do it. You have to do this, Ruth. Claim your husband back. Get him home and we can have our own vitamin press. His family are exhausted and have done all they can, so we're all in agreement here. Get him home. The hospital post over crateloads of IV vitamins and charge him for telephone consultations. It's worth it just to see a light in his eyes. Isn't it?

Back in North Cottage, my vitamin press is messy with labels lost somewhere three jars deep. I am mainlining magical pink mixtures of vitamins right into my husband's arm. His veins are pumped but he's still miserable. Tap out those air bubbles because they might kill him. I run between husband and babies. I try my best but I can't fix things this way. My superhero costume is the wrong fit and that's when I fall face first in the gravel.

Things are moving too fast and Simon's footsteps are getting slower. I hear an almighty crash in the hallway and run out to find him folded on the floor like a half sandwich. He is lying face up on his back, with his legs underneath him the wrong way. I am afraid he's broken, but he's not broken. His legs have just stopped. I help him into the wheelchair that has been a shadow in the corner for weeks. It has been camouflaged with a colourful army of well-placed teddies.

Things are moving fast but now Simon can move fast too. I strap the baby to my front and two eager boys park themselves on Simon's lap. Let's get some tunes pumping. We are racing down ramps and footpaths with running wheels. Chubby hands are dancing. We can get Simon moving and hearts skip beats. I am strong and we gain momentum as I push from behind. I can push with everything I've got. This superhero costume fits just right. I'm fine. We're fine, but our new wheels don't fit in this place. It's time to put the call out to some superhero friends. Let's just pray they answer the call from up high. I hope they have decent costumes.

Truth or Dave

On good days we are beachcombers. Sorry souls are drawn to the sea. They come to the cove for solace and leave clues behind. Some days we are the best detectives who beachcomb and find every clue. There are treasures here. We find a cluster of stones left on a ledge. The stones are scrawled with fine-tip, delicate drawings of owls and animals. Who drew these? Can we keep them? This could be somebody's shrine, but maybe they were left to be found. My son hands me an owl stone so I can put it in my pocket. We only keep one and leave the rest.

Motor Neurone Disease is a tough name for chewing around in a child's mouth. They call it Meuron disease instead. 'Will Dadda ever move again?' they ask matter-of-factly. 'No, he will never ever move again,' I reply and that's the truth. 'Aww, really? He's still a good Dadda even though he can't move,' they shrug.

Today at the cove we are treasure hunters. Jack likes gnarled bits of wood and the tiniest rocks. Raife looks for heart-shaped stones. He gathers smooth round pebbles to take home and tie with string. He will glue on some googly eyes, turning them into pets. Arden seeks coloured sea glass and dismembered body parts like crab claws. Sadie stamps her foot for real actual pirate gold but will settle for sparkly stones or a fancy shell. Hunter chases dogs.

'He is my own secret doll Dadda,' sings Sadie in a semi-pirouette. She climbs up on the bed beside Simon to croon sweet nothings and secrets into his ear. 'Can I watch Care Bears on your TV, Dadda? Close your eyes, Momma, and wait.' Whisper. Will he say yes? Make a wish. Keep your eyes closed. YES says the computer voice. 'He said YES!' she shouts in endless surprise. 'He's such a good Dadda,' she laughs, twirling his fringe through her fingertips.

Treasures are waiting to be found. We climb the cove ledge and find two glass jars perched high up on the rocks. They are filled with rainwater and folded bits of paper. My five wild urchins circle the jars hungrily. Treasure! I don't want to disturb the jars. They could be somebody's wishes. A big label is on each jar. TRUTH, DARE. Curiosity takes over. It's a truth or dare game. The game is long over and soaked by time. Can we play? Let's play just once. We allow ourselves to pick one secret per jar. The truth jar asks in a childish scribble, 'Have you ever peed in the sea?' YES, we all nod bashfully.

The Dare jar says: 'Throw a rock at somebody.' NO says the mother with a firm headshake.

'I think I remember running on the grass with Dadda in North Cottage,' says ten-year-old Jack, 'But I wish I remembered his voice. When I was little I used to point the TV remote at you, Momma, and pretend to turn your sound down.'

Sometimes, on rare beachcomber days, a man with bagpipes marches up and down the ledge blasting gutsy melodies that shake my bones. I dive off the steps to the sound of bagpipes into sunlit sparkled water. My tribe of children whoop from the shore. They throw their shoes to climb rocks barefoot. On good days we are scavengers gone wild.

'Will I ever get Meuron disease?' asks Raife with a twisty face.

'No, you will never ever get Meuron disease,' I reply. He walks around for a week with a limp and I get called into school. I find him in the sick bay with a worried face.

'Hey, guess what!' I cry with Christmas cheer. 'All of the doctors and scientists did some tests on Dadda's blood and do you know what they said? None of us will ever *ever* get Meuron disease. They promised.'

'Is that true?' falters Raife.

'*Truth,*' I nod firmly.

'My foot feels a lot better,' he admits.

'Let's run on the beach,' I suggest.

Children are like truth detectives. They hunt for it without mercy. I envy my children their truth when mine is space-bound to the moon in swirly grey shadows. There is no truth, only feelings. Can you see the moon's face? Sometimes I can, but the shapes keep changing. Feelings shift moment to moment and truth moves along with them. Stay true to your own feelings. That's the best I can hope for.

Arden can't remember but he doesn't say a word. He quietly places a framed photo by his bed of his dadda cuddling him when he was one. Rings of rolled fat reach up towards his dad's face and Simon is laughing.

They don't like it when he leaves the house. The noisy air mattress is laid bare and there's a big empty wheelchair space. 'Where's Dadda?' whines Hunter when Simon and the nurses are gone. I just want to whirl around in my underwear and leave the bathroom door wide open, but the kids are freaking out. 'I . . . miss . . . my . . . Dadda,' wails Hunter between tearful gasping gulps. 'We don't like it when Dadda's not here,' they all whinge.

They may not remember but I do. Some days the truth slaps hard. Most days I wake with a gasp. Who am I? What place is this and how did I get here? Who is this man in my house who can't move? Where is my Simon who pinches my waist with a cheeky smile?

My children are truth detectives and some days I can't keep up. On these days the air is gloomy. The sky is a heavy grey jumper with no air holes. I feel like I haven't slept when

I have. My limbs are so weary I could lie down on the ground and let leaves cover me. I am married to a bearded stranger with intense eyes. The kids deserve better than a mother who feels like this. I don't want to damage my children. That is my only truth on these dark days.

I stand before a sparkling sea and turn to see a gull on a rock. He looks so solid. Waves are lapping at the lower step and sucking my feet in swirls. The gull is on more solid ground than me. Michelle says we just have to ride the wave. Ride the wave and remember that a wave came before you. Even if you've missed it, another one is coming up right behind you. Waves go on for ever, so just go with it. She is such a lovely hippie.

'Come in here and meet my Dadda,' says Raife to his schoolmate with a shifty grin. 'He has Meuron disease and a computer voice and he can't move. It's OK! Come in and say hello. Go on! I dare you.' Raife is having fun with a glint in his eye. This is pure entrapment. He just wants to gauge his friend's reaction. When meeting Simon most kids have eyes like saucers. Some are curious and ask questions. Others run from the room yelling that it's too weird. 'It's just my Dadda,' says Raife with a shrug. I want to protect him but the great joke is that he is protecting me. Through five pairs of eyes, I see that Dadda is just Dadda. Things are what they are. TRUTH.

Some good days at the cove start off feeling bad. It's windy and cold until our feet hit the sand and we dare to run. It's warmer than we thought and nobody else is here. This beach is ours and we claim full ownership. We will collect stones for Dadda. I only wish we could hand the whole cove to Simon so he could put it in his pocket. It starts lashing rain and we just don't care. We are whooping and laughing and climbing and swimming. We will continue to beachcomb, hunt, and scavenge for clues. Treasures are left to be found and we know this is true. Sorry souls do what they can to survive, so just go with it. I dare you.

Dancing

I fell in love with some dancing hands. You don't expect to fall in love with hands. Simon would speak words and his fingers would follow suit. His hands drew invisible letters in thin air. His fingers moved frantically to tune in his fine talk. Those hands were the dance beat weaving together the entire earblasting soundtrack. I drank in his eyes, his hands, his face, all moving together in some kind of fast symphony. This was by far my favourite song. I could listen to this tune on repeat. I could dance along for ever.

Two souls swing together and attempt to share a life. Often these souls sing to wildly different tunes. My soul is most likely a cheesy Abba song, rhyming words with a hearty refrain. Simon loves hectic jazz, indie misery and booming opera. Hell is a place on earth that listens to Leonard Cohen around the dinner table. The horror. Simon would love that. I would have to put my cutlery down quietly and jump out the nearest window.

Simon's blue eyes now dart around a computer screen. Letters in square boxes get highlighted as he settles on a phrase. He picks words from a predictive text database. Sentences are formed. His hands and face are motionless. Fingers with long clean nails lie limply on propped cushions. The dance is slow and careful and full of wrong moves. I stand beside him shifting from foot to foot. I wait for his words as patiently as I can, but children are yelling to be rescued from lost socks, unwiped bottoms, toys on a high shelf and unopened bananas. The dance stops and starts so often I get twitchy. I linger on his beautiful eyes and attempt to change my pace. I beg with my brain to please not let our dance disconnect, but it does. His words can't come fast enough and it's just too damn hard. Shouts from the children have reached operatic crescendos. With heavy shoulders, I leave the room.

We danced together at our wedding and the truth is that we were terrible dancers. Our rhythm was off so we just clung together and giggled. Our parents jived around us in perfect harmony to the sounds of Mama Cass. We laughed and looked on in admiration. Our lives lay long and languidly ahead of us. There was plenty of time to get the moves right. Five years later I danced with a friend at my brother's wedding and he explained to me patiently that one person has to lead. Then he spun me around the floor in perfect circles. I learned that lesson too late for Simon to spin me around a dance floor.

*

Every year since MND, Simon's aunt buys us tickets to the Opera. Wexford Opera House is a grand and glorious place of smooth circular wood and warm lights. It is a black tie event filled with opulent old ladies draped in furs and diamonds. Simon wears a tux and his nurse, Adam, positions a colourful cravat discreetly over the tracheostomy at his throat. The air pipe snakes secretly under his black jacket, back to the crooning ventilator behind his wheelchair. We drive for two hours to get there and smiling ushers lead us in. The fine old ladies elbow past the wheelchair in a scramble for the lift. In a comical dance, they fall over his wheels and beat us to the elevator doors. Old age earns you a one-way ticket to outrageously selfish behaviour. I just love these crazy old dears.

The lights go down and Simon gets lost in the swell of the strong orchestral swarm. Tears gather in his eyes and I squeeze his hand. I think it's all great but secretly I'm more of a *Wicked* girl and Simon knows this. Adam is with us. Adam is young and perpetually hungry. I warned him to eat before we left because the Opera outing is a long day. We will stop for chips on the way home. I spend most of the Opera daydreaming about future chips and the time I saw *Wicked* with my mum and sister and cried my eyes out.

I fell in love with Simon's dancing hands and now they don't move. For a long time his left hand had just a tiny twitch left.

The kids called it his 'imping'. In bed beside him, I would slip my hand under his palm when we were watching movies and his imping would dance along. One day or another it finally faded and just stopped. Simon's fingers can no longer tune in his words, but my love for those hands still lingers. I want to keep the nails cut down because they grow too long. He gets scared that I will cut too far to the quick. I rub them and hold them and rest them on cushions. Children and nurses slip hand warmers under them when he asks. The dance has left his hands in a permanent disconnect. I can drink in the deep of those eyes, but dammit, those hands had a fine sexy beat. I miss that dance so much.

I am standing in a chipper in the town of Ferns in fine Opera clothes. My eyes are tired from driving. Pretending to be grown-ups is how I describe the Opera trip to my husband. A television screen flashes above my head in this bright Italian chipper and it's pumping out a loud dance beat. I scrunch up my toes in tight woman shoes. I am squirming in my fake fur jacket. The dance beat is teasing me. I look up, and on the screen a young girl in a tan leotard is dancing wildly around a tiny room. This girl is twisting and throwing and bending her body around a confined space. She is a wild prepubescent animal, caged and raging with schizophrenic fake smiles. My tired eyes are transfixed and I am filled with dread.

Pretending to be grown-ups isn't funny any more. I don't want to be this person wearing a fancy lady's dress. My shoes are killing me. I want to run around the room screaming at the walls and beating them with fists. I need to move, bend, drag, twist my body away from all this. I'm not ready to be bodiced into old age. The dance beat is tearing up my soul. Opera years are piling up like old ladies over Simon's wheels. Their fur coats will smother me before we make the lift doors. I fucking hate the Opera. It's not a joke. The wildness in me is very much alive. I take my warm bag of chips and thank the man politely. Adam and I eat our chips silently in the car with Simon asleep in the back and then we drive home.

I can't stop thinking about the girl in the leotard. Puffy eyed with weary feet, I show her to the children next morning over our cornflakes. Six of us huddle around my laptop. 'She is totally freaky,' says Raife. 'She's dancing!' squeals Sadie. 'Turn it up!' yells Jack. Suddenly we are all wordlessly throwing shapes around the kitchen with the girl. Sadie swirls her hands in the air. Hunter jiggles. Raife runs on the spot and Jack pumps fists. Arden falls to the floor in full break-dance. I throw my body in with them, laughing my ass off.

We could dance this way for ever as long as we keep the door closed. A nurse comes in and the kids self-consciously stop. I keep on kicking it and they all start up again. Keep on dancing, keep moving I tell them and everything will be OK. It has to be. I won't give up on the dance, because if I do we are all doomed. My Opera-weary muscles stretch out and I dream of a nowhere somewhere space with fast beats. This is the place where Simon and I are finally spinning around a dance floor. We move in perfect synch and his hands are still dancing.

Watered

Good friends know how to keep you well watered. By these watering standards our friends Daragh and Cath are good friend superheroes. It makes perfect sense that Daragh is also a water engineer. Cath and I had our first babies together. Jack and Theo were born in the same month. We would park chubby parcels between us in coffee shops and talk endlessly over jammy scones.

Before MND we were faraway neighbours in Greystones. Daragh and Simon embraced DIY. Days were endless. They did man stuff like pave pathways and rotavate garden soil. Cath showed me how to pot plants properly so they stayed alive. Then they went and emigrated to Australia, we moved to North Cottage and Simon bloody well got MND. Endless days were over.

I have always had a problem with plants. It is never as simple as just keeping them watered. Watered or not, they defy every care I give them and just die. At Christmas red poinsettias go crispy. Summer blooms hang their dead heads before I get near to deadheading them. Orchids are a conundrum and even cactuses look sad and shrivelled. My mother-in-law gave me a lemon tree once that filled me full of dread.

Marian is good with plants. She breezes through our home quietly saving tiny green souls. Orchids bloom by her hand and lemons hang fat. I love this woman. 'You don't water them enough and then you overwater them,' sighs Marian, which is way too complex a notion for me. Love them too little or love them too much. Either way is not enough. Watering just got far too technical. I nod in careful agreement and then leave her to it.

When MND started to take over North Cottage, I knew in my heart what we needed. Simon had been diagnosed less than a year but was already in a wheelchair. We were soaked in vitamins and lost hope. The boys needed to see us laugh and be brave, hugging hard onto the life that we had.

I craved a Mad Hatter's tea party and some cracked plates. Playing things too safe would swamp us. I calmly told myself what we had to do. Dive into sparkly sunshine and find the good friends who first taught us the superhero code. Get back into the light. Follow Daragh and Cath to Australia with these new wheels.

I feel nervous watching the attendants push my husband down the aisle of the plane on narrow, tiny wheels. Baby Arden is too big for the bassinet cot on the wall but my arms get so tired, I wedge him in there anyway. He sleeps soundly with a dented head. Jack and Raife shout the eleven-hour flight with loud headphone voices. I choreograph an aeroplane dance around all of them, involving nappies, wipes, bottles, toilet trips, snacks, naps and cartoons. Not knowing he can't walk, fellow passengers scowl at stationary Simon like he's the biggest asshole father of all time. We giggle together in the heat of their glares. Two souls take flight in this plane fuelled up on adventure.

Ironically, we get watered in one of the driest places on the planet. If Ireland is overcast and brooding, Perth is all scorched earth and sunlight. It feels free from moisture and heavy thought. The dampness and cloying doubt get burnt away. We drive through dry winds under blue skies. Smooth red roads and roundabouts circle our days. So many suburban signs slip by with a sea breeze and a sense of space. Oh yes, I like it in Perth. And Daragh and Cath are here to greet us.

Perth is such a parched piece of land, the government gives grants for fake plastic grass on front lawns. We learn a new watering word in Perth. The word is reticulation. Reticulation is the complex system of sprinklers set on a timer that folks use to water their gardens. Real lawns are so neat, lush and systematically watered that they look fake anyway.

Reticulation sprinklers are only turned on at designated times of the day. It's a system that saves all of Perth's tiny green souls.

I am determined to get Simon well watered in Perth. I watch the sprinklers go off in sequence. Just keep his soul saturated. You can do this, Ruth. Get up, jump, skip, dodge the dark looks, keep him talking and his face in sunshine. I have arms that can carry, push, pull and heave. Baby Arden is strapped to my body while Jack and Raife sit on Simon's lap. We walk the smooth streets this way. Simon's wheelchair is a Daddy-shaped children's buggy. He wraps his arms around soft boy skin. They whoop and laugh as I push them at a run and we freewheel under bright blue skies. Simon grows to love his new wheels. Wheels can be so lovable in a place with good footpaths.

We are totally invincible. I don't even feel tired. Fold that wheelchair up and throw it in the boot. Heave Simon into the front seat on a plank of wood and let's drive. We have the freedom to go where we please. Broken baby nights and physical days are easy because we are high on the achievement of really living again.

Systems can help Simon, and Daragh and Cath design a system of fun. We lower him by hoist into the swimming pool, arms adorned with three layers of floatie bands. He bobs around with a face full of bliss. There are trips to the museum and windy parks. We lift him together in a king's chair and lower him on to green manicured grass. We eat eggs, avocado and feta and drink the best damn coffee in the land. This place is all sea breeze and beach toes, dazzling blues and dry heat. I think I might love it here.

Daragh does bombies with the kids in the pool as Simon floats around. I watch my boys get physical with man-boy play and it is wonderful to watch them go wild. Daragh wrestles them with hairy bear hugs. He brews beer and bakes lemon tarts. His engineering brain embraces such skills with ease. He patiently explains pipes, manholes and reticulation systems to the kids. The boys dance naked through sprinklers circling the grass. Their milky white bottoms are mini moons catching the sun.

In Australia I get superhero clothes. I literally dance in my pants. Mornings are too hot to wear anything but knickers as I clean the swimming pool. The boys hang loose in nappies, sun hats and rubber Croc shoes studded with badges. We throw the kids and their plastic shoes in the bath at the end of each day to soak away the desert dust. Knickers and flip-flops will do me just fine. I become obsessed with the two funnest domestic tasks known to mankind: cleaning the pool and hanging out washing. Clothes reduce to hard husks after only an hour's drying.

Cath is a creative soul who cooks, plants, knits and sews. Throughout our stay she is making a patchwork quilt. Each square is a letter of the alphabet. Every morning she arrives at the door with an easy smile and another letter. She sits and sews with the kids while I help Simon get to the bathroom and get dressed. Functional carer duties are easier to cope with if you say them quickly and get them done fast. Don't dwell on the details, even in your own mind. I have never had help like this. Cath makes it feel so simple. She sews us back together with the steely calm motion of her needle and thread.

Perth is a reticulation system all of its own. Sprinklers surround us. They spray soft water on our sorry souls. Endless rounds of sun, heat, movie dates, fast sunsets, blackout blinds, plastic Christmas trees, pizza in the park, swimming pools, scorched car seats, morning coffee, complex train tracks, children in the fridge, wees on the floor, cockroaches in the dishwasher, demonic flies, Simon's first movie script, tears, sex, love and AIRCON busy our days. All of it is good. We are well watered and start to get steady.

Sometimes Simon goes drinking with Daragh. They come home late, giggling and smelling of beer bubbles. Daragh drunkenly helps Simon back into our double bed. I roll over one night and wake to find Daragh calmly straddling my husband to prop him up with pillows. 'Sorry we woke you,' they both say. This kind of bizarre help quenches my soul.

It is in Perth that I notice the sea for the first time. It sings stories to me of a forgotten wildness I once forged as a child. My five siblings and I spent feral beach days on the shores of Co. Donegal. The Slidey Beach, the Secret Beach, the Big Beach – there were so many beaches, we claimed ownership of golden sand and christened them with names. In Perth the sand is a startling white. Men heave and tanned torsos strain, as Daragh and his friends carry Simon down to sit at the water's edge. Waves are large enough to eat small toddlers here and Cath points up to a bright yellow rescue helicopter circling the sky. 'That means a shark's in the water,' she explains. We paddle tentatively near wet sand, a watchful eye eternally trained skywards. Wildness be damned, we mostly stick to the pool for swimming.

I feel alive every day. The sun paints a happy face on my heart. The ocean air empties heads and heals broken hearts. Arden is nearing his first birthday. His blue eyes look out to sea and his face creases into the wind. I wonder about his view through those long lashes. I recall that childlike feeling of possibilities. I had forgotten the simplicity of an empty, happy head.

There are some dark days in the sunshine. In our favourite seaside cafe, Simon begins to struggle when lifting his coffee cup. Sometimes he sits so quietly, just staring at walls. I watch his spirit flicker like a candle left in a draught. I love him. I want him to have a happy life with us. That view of possibilities through Arden's eyes should be shared with the man who helped make him. Simon sometimes sits so still that I know he is very far away from me. I don't know how it must feel to be him and it scares me to my bones.

Are superheroes allowed to get scared? Maybe knickers

are not suitable superhero attire. They are lacking in basic armour. Some days I park my car at the beach and just cry. In Perth they have designated dog beaches designed for dog-walkers and closet criers. Crying empties you out so you can fill up again. There is no denying that I am drawn to the beach and the sea. Dog Beach is a place where my mind runs free and grieves.

Systems can keep you well watered but sometimes they feel like a load of fake grass. I am not good with plants. I overwater. I worry that I am an equally bad friend. Sickness makes us crouch selfishly in a tight circle with our immediate own. Empathy for friends is lost. We just don't have room. Superhero friends gave us their car, their house and their hearts. Some day I will repay you, I tell Cath. I have woven these people around my heart and I will never let them go.

The time comes to return to Ireland and we have to let them go. A six-week holiday turned to six months is the furthest we could stretch. It is March and Jack needs to start school in September. I don't want to go back. Black clouds are gathering and there is no bargaining with them. Simon's arms are so weak he strains to lift them up and his voice is getting quieter. They bundle him on to the plane where his wheels feel so confined again. The freewheeling days are over.

The sense of dread feels endless. As we descend into dimly

lit cloud and dark green fields, I have a horrible realisation. My superhero costume has slipped. Humans are the trickiest of plants. Over- or underwatering may yield the same results. I am no superhero. Nothing I can do will stop MND or save my husband.

Fear

I am not afraid of dying and I never have been. This may be the truth or maybe it just feels that way. As a teenager, I sat in the family car en route to a holiday in France. My parents were in their *Riverdance* phase. They blared Celtic beats on repeat as we drove down a monotonous straight road through a forest. Ireland had just hosted Eurovision and I had finished my Leaving Cert.

Enormous trees slipped by in quick succession. Tall perpendicular trunks dazzled me; they stretched for miles in every direction. The moving car spun trees like a zoetrope while I stared out the window. I was overwhelmed with a feeling of insignificance in the vastness of a spinning world.

This existential tree moment is the closest I've ever come to fearing death. Possibly it was just the *Riverdance* music, though. The collective sound of so many Irish dancing feet still freaks me out. They are just so damned synchronised.

Perhaps chronic daydreamers don't fear death because we are used to slipping away. Death could be just another dreamy escape. Michelle drove up the Wicklow hills in her jeep recently and parked to lie on the roof for some stargazing. The night sky was so bright that she raised her hands right up into it. She could feel herself floating away. It was exactly like swimming in stars, she said.

Aifric describes her brain like a scene from *James and the Giant Peach*. Her cluttered, chaotic thoughts are the hundreds of birds on strings dragging her peachy brain over the ocean. Swimming in the sea plunges that peach so deep in cold that the birds disperse and scatter. Her brain breaks free from heavy thought.

It feels like arrogance not to fear death when Simon lives so fearfully close to it. What the hell do I know in my dumb healthy body? He is Dylan Thomas raging against the dying of the light. This burning rage is not something I can fully understand. He cannot seem to contemplate his own departure. The real problem with rage is the burning part. There is no peace, and burns can really hurt.

I have often felt the thrill of floating far from here. It happened deep-sea diving in Australia once at the Great Barrier Reef. My boyfriend at the time was a cautious diver and I had never tried it before. The underwater world was a revelation. Cartoon colours sang in my brain. I joined a shoal of fish and happily tried to swim away. Any deeper and the bends would have taken me for sure. I was pulled back by an ankle grab and reluctantly returned to the surface.

Not fearing death should never be confused with a need. I have no desire for it, but death just won't shut up. Sharing your home with illness means it cannot be ignored. Hello Death. MND brought you to the party and you are both sneaky gatecrashers. Neither of you got invited but I will keep my manners in check. It's rude to ignore house guests and impossible when they are so rowdy.

The sea and the universe are breathing, says Michelle. Sometimes, if you're lucky, you can breathe in time with them. She sat on a mountain once in America looking down on a valley far below. She sat very still and was so high up that it felt like she left her body. The trees and the sky and the mountains were all part of the same thing. Michelle was just part of it too. She was breathing in time with the universe. It is worth pointing out again that Michelle is a total hippie.

Simon breathes in time to a machine. Fear surrounds the plugs, pipes, power cuts and the countless malfunctions that could end his life. I love him so I don't like that he is afraid. I hold his hand and doubt he will ever speak to death or stop being scared of it. And yet he is the bravest man. In some ways, Dylan Thomas really sucks.

When you sea-swim in the depths of winter with only a

rubber hat for cover, a funny thing happens. Stay in the water too long and you don't feel like coming back out. The cold seeps so deep into your bones that your brain begins to hear an ocean song calling you. This song is something way better than *Riverdance*.

Dreams and I float side by side in such seas. I stare at the horizon hungrily. My body feels the urge to keep relaxing and just drift away. A profound peace comes over me and I could become part of this wave for ever. I wonder if this is what dying feels like. A gentle thought slips by, within close enough range for me to hear it. My children might need me. With wobbly limbs, I reluctantly climb out of the water. I am stumbling like a gangly foal.

What is this strange magic of the sea? I dive into a dancing, breathing ocean. The cold casts this spell of fearlessness that defies life and death. The only thing cold cannot defy is the seaweed. I am petrified of the stuff. Tangles of it make me scream like a little girl. My mind wants to merge with the ocean, despite seaweed, fear, and maybe the odd jellyfish.

Lots of things scare me but death just isn't one of them. Along with seaweed, there are spiders and earwigs and heights of any kind. I got vertigo so badly as a kid climbing a tree that my uncle had to reach up and rescue me. I was clinging with my eyes closed to the very lowest branch.

As a child I was too afraid to jump. I cringed in the corners of Portsalon pier in Donegal. Younger kids hurtled past me into swirly waters below. Even in a life jacket, I still couldn't do it. The fear is still with me, but these days I jump anyway. I have always been the world's biggest ninny. Survival simply stepped in. Circumstance has struck me into some kind of groundhog day sea swimming time loop.

The fearless spell will last just as long as you stay in the ocean. It drags at your limbs near the water's edge. Back in the busy world, the brain gasps and quickly forgets. That's why we will plunge again and again. We are drawn back here by the pure romance of breathing in perfect synch. I share this magic with my Tragic Wives, Michelle and Aifric. We linger at the cove and dive in.

Kicking Cars

What do you do on dark days? How do you dance when everything you could possibly want comes exactly as it's being taken away? MND is like water torture, slowly drip-drip-dripping. A tiny nerve ending, a small piece of strength, gets stolen every single day.

Bleached goodbyes in Perth seem far away in cold Greystones where we wonder how we can ever get used to Ireland again, we look to the grey skies and feel stumped. Dirty roads, dirty cars says a two-year-old Raife. Yes, my love, our world looks smudgy.

When superheroes lose their powers it never ends well. They get dramatically destroyed. I imagine exploding in company. I could self-combust at the supermarket in a fine sticky mess over mild chats about all the rain we've been having.

Why can't I wake those nerves up? Shake them back to life? Slap him in the face? Home from Perth I get so angry.

MAKE IT STOP WHY CAN'T YOU MAKE IT STOP. STAY WITH US, WE LOVE YOU. WE NEED YOU, WE DON'T WANT TO BE HERE WITHOUT YOU. Then I cry from a very dark place and fall deep.

North Cottage got flooded so we fixed the roof and put it on the market. A brief glance, a shivery goodbye, we set forth for a house in Greystones and the glow of living among people.

Simon's arms are so weak he is upgraded to a power wheelchair. He whizzes down corridors, lifting carpets up like waves. He drives the boys by himself in the middle of the road right through traffic. His wheels form fantastic fuck off fingers to the terrible footpaths. My heart sings but it's a warbly sort of song. I used to grip the back of his chair. My push is no longer needed. I wave goodbye to the bond and feel one step closer to loneliness.

Back in Greystones there is so much rain. It's hard being back where we lived first married. That life was all cliff walks, coffees and casual strolls. This place is confusing and cross.

'I wish that Dadda could walk like other Daddas,' Jack wails at four years of age, 'I want to cry for ever'. Then he makes a good stab at it. I know this cry so well. It's from the deepest place. It stirs you up so you think your insides will spill out. It's a disgusting physical mess of a cry that retches out the darkest parts. 'It's not FAIR,' he cries and I know it's not.

To see my boy cry like this makes me angry. But not just

one boy. Two tinier hearts weep and roar in the wings; his loyal back-up singers. They understand even less but know for sure that it's shit.

What do you do? You want your head to blow up in bright sparks because that is what feels should happen. You can't curl into a ball in a dark room because children are crying with empty cups. They are fighting for toast. It has to be you because there is nobody else to do it, and without a superhero suit you think, what is the point?

An angry brain screams fast, angry thoughts. There is no hope for these beautiful boys. They will end up in rehab or drug addicts or on mystery milk cartons because their mother got shouting mad and their father stared at walls from his wheelchair and then died. Is this where we're going because there's nowhere else to go? His arms will stop working and he won't be able to talk. I will want to die myself because it's too large to bear the weight of it. We will have orphan Oliver Twist children. Oh please, sir, I want no more.

Froths of anger loom largely over every donation of help. Say hello to the 'How are things?' brigade. I don't know how to answer. Away from Perth, the help offered just never fits quite right. Nobody speaks my language. I sit in Tesco's car park crying and it's no Dog Beach.

We drive a comical wheelchair car. It's Postman Pat's van painted blue. I drive slowly so Simon doesn't get hurt by the bumps. He sits high in the back while his three boys fight and chat in the middle.

We all jump at the howl of a car horn. A low green convertible cuts me off at a T-junction. It's just another road rage driver beeping us in traffic. We meet them every day, but today something breaks. The green beast stops at a red light up ahead and I pull up behind him. My body goes calm. 'Back in a second,' I bark at the boys.

What do you do with the pain, when you're world weary and really angry at the same time? I have banged my head against walls. It bled and I saw stars. I have stared at my scrawny arms and imagined red gashes slashing fat blue veins. I have crumpled to the floor, hiding behind kitchen presses, hugging my knees for dear life. I have drunk and smoked, overeaten, undereaten, all the foods both good and bad. I have fought shallow breaths till my lungs burst, gasped till I'm numb, laughed till I cried and cried manic laughing tears.

I march up to the driver's window and a middle-aged man glances out. 'I was driving slowly because my husband is in a wheelchair,' I shout. 'Maybe you didn't see the big wheelchair sticker?' He waves me away and puts up the window. 'You're a very rude man,' I shout, more loudly this time. He won't look at me and I decide to kick the shit out of his car. I keep kicking and kicking until the light goes green and he speeds off again. I am breathing heavily but feel amazingly calm. An onlooker on the footpath waves, cheers and gives me a thumbs-up.

Angry tears have drowned me in dark pits. Buried in fits of black panic, there is no starry sky. I have picked my nails raw and bitten my hand so hard it broke skin, leaving toothy scar smiles. I have done all this and yet I am still here. I have never fully broken. Our dark world now fills me with the urge to break stuff. I want to break everything and just smash this shit up.

Returning to our Postman Pat van, I click quietly into my seat belt. The boys sit with open mouths. 'Momma, what did you do THAT for?' asks Jack. 'Sorry, love,' I reply. 'That man was just a fucking asshole.' I still feel calm but my hands are shaking so badly I can barely turn the ignition. 'You said the F word!' says Jack in delight.

'Yep, your momma most definitely said the F word,' says Simon and we laugh as the ignition key finally turns. The engine revs a mighty Postman Pat roar. Momentarily, this destroyed superhero feels remarkably fine.

Food

Love is glorious and so is food. Put the two together and dreams can come true. Food surrounds many of my fondest memories with Simon. Our love came wrapped in a burrito. His hand on a coffee cup made my heart flutter. When we first met I lost my appetite, but I got it back quickly enough. My soul was soon hungry beyond words.

A boy with a big voice impressed me at a party once. He spoke loudly with lofty principles on vegetarianism. 'Take an animal's life with your own hands if you want. But unless you're willing to kill a chicken, I don't think you should eat one.' His words stayed with me and I stopped eating meat. The boy was Simon but I barely knew him back then. By the time we dated years later, we were both devoted to lentils.

The rush of first love brings Mexican food rituals every Sunday. Light-headed and spent, we hop in taxis that transport us to tasty *huevos rancheros*. We make moon eyes at each other in candlelit restaurants over pasta. Soul explosions and mouth-watering tastes stir together and we are still starving.

I watch our four-year-old twins eat their dinner in unison with finely tuned forks. Meals are a shared symphony. Sadie likes the pasta and Hunter prefers the sausage. One wordlessly assists the other so they can pick both plates clean. My family introduced Simon to Indian food. He accidentally ate some lime pickle and his face went alarmingly red. My four brothers clapped him on the back. When the teasing applause ceased, they were all invested as brothers. Both our families love nothing more than to bond loudly over good food and lashings of wine.

Our love got served up on a fine veggie platter. We insisted on a vegetarian wedding. Belligerent meat-eaters grumbled and growled for steak by the bar. We danced badly but groovily in the knowledge that no bird was sacrificed at the altar of our big day. Our Italian honeymoon made pasta ribbons of my heart. Love, mozzarella and linguine mixed with rapid heartbeats.

When the kids are small we have nights away in hotels. Simon hangs duvets between the cots and the double bed to soundproof our three boys to sleep. We sit on the big bed watching movies and gleefully order as much room service as possible. Hotels exist for lovemakers to lock themselves in bed ordering food. Isn't that their purpose?

*

'Thanks for making me a boiled egg,' says eight-year-old Raife. 'I feel so graceful.' 'Do you mean grateful?' I ask. 'Eh, no, I think I mean graceful,' he replies. I will forever draw a giant scribbly loveheart around Simon, his talk and good dinners. I just cannot separate, love, food and the sound of his sexy voice. The three combined are God-given grace.

Back from Australia, food started to become functional. Simon's voice got quieter. His mouth slid around slurred words. Fear formed around food and manageable bite-sized chunks. Chewing took time. Choking fits chased us around dinner. Giant smoothies were easier. We had bucket-sized Starbucks cups with big straws.

When appetite dwindled, another bond took its place. The carer–patient bond may not sound so sexy but it is stronger than the urge to eat.

By the time Simon landed in hospital with pneumonia, we were so silently in tune I could almost read his thoughts. My hands knew where to lift. A mere glance of his eyes could tell me where it hurt and how I could help. I stayed on a makeshift bed in his hospital room, pummelling his chest to assist each strained cough. I had left the three boys with my mother to live like this. I don't remember eating. Perhaps there were some coffees and cardboard sandwiches. The important thing was to just keep Simon breathing. My hands could help him as long as they kept their focus.

When they whisk him away, I haven't really slept for three days. I have forgotten all about my own children. I am like an extension of him, in tune with every need and he can't breathe. 'Help me, Ruth, help,' he pleads and nobody can help him but me. My hands are keeping him alive. I am on top of him screaming as his trolley is pushed towards ICU, pushing, pushing, pushing his lungs for air. They have to pull me off him and I cling with a vice grip. The door of the ICU slams shut and I am left outside on a bench.

He can stay alive by my hand. Without my hands I am sure he has just died. He needs me to breathe but the superhero me is spent. My arms are so weak from pressing his chest that I can barely lift them. I think Simon just died, I say. His life is now in the hands of others. I think of my children. Numbness and anguish rest side by side. It's a feeling of pure relief.

Simon doesn't die but he is put on a ventilator. The three hospital months that follow are blurry, punctuated only by the food we eat. The sight of their dad in ICU with tubes leaves the boys bewildered. They are delighted by the giant bowls of jelly and ice cream the nurses pile upon them. We sit in the brightly lit coffee shop munching mini packets of Cheerio hoops. We cross the road for better coffee at Starbucks and slices of cake. Food is something we recognise and it gives the day shape.

I am hungry all the time but I can't seem to taste. Exhaustive planning meetings take place at the hospital in the hope that we'll get Simon home. I sit with his family. The ICU has no windows. This is impossible to comprehend. The hospital mediator has the slowest voice of all time. I want to curl up on the floor and maybe eat a Pot Noodle.

I return home late at night to watch movies and eat Indian takeaway alone. It is tasteless. I am beyond tears and exhaustion. Simon gets a tube put in his stomach so he doesn't have to eat at all. A tracheostomy at his throat means he can speak but only with a special valve. His voice is croaky slow and harder to understand, so he's learning to use an eye gaze computer. He will come home with a team of five nurses alternating 12-hour night and day shifts. They wield big syringes to fill his stomach with a sticky sweet food supplement. It smells like cheap plastic ice cream, the kind that hurts your teeth.

I visit the Asian superstore that Sadie calls the silly shop. We're not sure why. It reminds me of my veggie-flavoured Hindu-loving heart. Blocks of paneer cheese, bindis and bags of rice surround beautiful brown-eyed women and grumpy shuffling men. Love was once made of lentils, chana masala, fifty varieties of noodles, hot counters of crispy bhajis, butter biscuits, vanilla-flavoured Coca-Cola and – oh, bless us – the silly shop just makes my silly heart sing.

The only things making sense in this new world are meal-times and children have to be fed. I mechanically cook meals but don't remember tasting them. I visit my parents for dinner and feel lonely with my separate veggie portion. Something primal in me wants to share the same food as them, cook the beast, tear it apart and break bread. Lentils have no love in them since the ICU.

To hell with the animals when you live in hell. I have wolfish survival instincts and they are harshly tit for tat. Simon is forced to live like this and he can almost die like that. In the grand scheme of things, fuck the chickens. Life seems so tenuous and sacrificial. These hands would gladly take a chicken's life. Let me wring some scrawny necks. My soul is starving and I need to eat.

Twins

There are five children in my house. Who put them here? I am tripping up over a dog, a cat and a hamster who bites hands. Clutter and chaos are here too. They are close friends who bring me the most calm. This is lucky, because they have me surrounded.

My childhood home always left me feeling oddly perplexed. I grew up knee deep in higgledy-piggledy. Where did six children and all the pets come from? Animals and babies crowded recklessly in corners. For years, an upturned cushion hid the melted hole where my brother had tried to set fire to the sofa.

My dad ran his doctor's surgery from the house. He had six willing receptionists. 'I'm not here!' he'd yell. We all grew up with impeccable phone manners. My mother had to wade through odd shoes and Dinky cars flung from the stairwell, to answer the front door. My poor parents had to barricade themselves with a baby gate just to eat their dinner. Their plates were perched on knees for a hasty ten minutes while children pawed at the gate like zombies. I take pride in chaos because for some mad reason it means happy children.

Simon grew up in a tidy home with two sisters. He had bathrooms where the towel colours matched the shampoo bottles. Chaos never came as naturally to him but he went along with mine. He knew all about growing up with love. I casually constructed sculptures of odds and ends on counter tops. He would sweep them away like litter. I like to think we complemented each other and the result was happy balance.

I might just have a thing for babies. Animal or human, it doesn't really matter. Perhaps it's a kind of madness. I'm such a sucker for a cute face. 'She's got that look in her eye,' my friends will mutter. Hold on to your pets and babies. I might just steal one.

In our first Greystones home, just married, a stray cat took up residence in our backyard. She gave birth to five kittens. We kept one kitten, she had another litter and the cycle continued. Where did all these cats come from? I unwittingly became resident mad cat lady of our housing estate.

Growing up, we had lots of pets but our house leaned against a busy main road. So many cats sped through some fast cars and short lives. My mother would solve this conundrum by simply getting another pet.

Our cat went wild with the move to North Cottage. She

wandered far and left mouse guts by the half-door. Simon found her in the ditch one day with the life knocked right out of her. Her hair stood on end but her body had no marks. A fast lorry had swept her off her sturdy clawed feet. Even cat paws can't dodge a death that swift.

When a pet dies, there is an empty space left where they used to be. You no longer feel or hear them moving through your world. They are just gone. There's an empty cat bowl. The door of the cat house is left ajar. Death has come quickly, easily, as a matter of course. Dying is a brutally banal occurrence, like pouring the milk into your tea. A cat bed covered in hairs and some unopened tins in the press. It happens so quietly, definitely with no fuss and a cruel finality. All you have left is this sad echo of things.

We got busy soundproofing sad echoes. Our cat's nine lives were up, so we searched for a puppy. We drove to Wexford and found ourselves a basset hound. He bounded on to the lawn with his brothers and sisters, tripping up over his long ears. Our own babies couldn't have been cuter. It is love at first sight and we name him Pappy.

Simon came home from ICU on a ventilator and with 24-hour nursing care. My chaotic brain was no match for a hospital in my home.

Here is my husband back with tubes trailing out of him. Noisy suction machines and beeping ventilators bark loudly.

Fear dances in his eyes. My heart is breaking so I do the only thing I know how. I dump children on his lap and animals at his feet. Kids climb through pipes and wade through wires. Their chubby hands find his face. They play. Jack grabs the back of his wheelchair and Simon drags him around the floor. The room swells with peals of boy laughter.

It makes perfect sense to have another baby, because we still can. Practical discussions and questioning of doctors don't even come into it. For me this is survival the only way I know how. The making requires some manoeuvring with raised hospital beds and standing-up wheelchairs. Mind and body have to jump through some gymnastic hoops. But we managed.

Free from the windowless ICU, Simon has a new view. He is finishing the script for his first feature-length film, the one he started before MND and toiled over in Australia. He plans to be the first director with MND to ever make a movie. He might write a book as well. Fast-forward action flips to floods of tears in a heartbeat, but he's trying so hard I can feel it. It rallies us together like a team. His bravery builds bonds that feel unbreakable.

Bring on the chaos, but I wasn't expecting two of them. At the 20-week scan, we want to avoid the element of surprise. Is the baby a boy or a girl we ask nervously. 'Which one, because you know there's two of them,' says the nice lady. 'You're joking,' I reply. 'I'm not joking,' she bristles, clearly insulted at the idea. I have no concept of twins. There are none in my family. If it's two more boys I might jump out that window, I think. Simon's eyes get wider. 'Twin number one is a girl,' she says and we both burst into tears. Benedict, nurse of the mighty Tuc crackers, is with us too. His face beams rays of sunshine.

I've had a terrible hunger. Twins! Perhaps it was all the damn chicken. They are born by Caesarean with Simon and his wheels by my side . This feels like some kind of Caesarean birth party. I could swear that nurse has balloons under her scrubs. They let our family in straight afterwards for tears and photos. We have two new doll-sized babies, Sadie and Hunter. Simon can't reach for them so I wedge them in the crook of his arms wrapped up like baby burritos.

Simon has a new team around him and so do I. My mother moves in for a month and we share night feeds. The twins pull everyone together with new purpose. Simon's mother and sisters share rotas minding the boys. Friends who don't know about the chicken leave so many spinach and ricotta bakes by our front door we turn green.

We think that, as people, our death will be more profound, more meaningful, more dramatic than the death of a pet. But it won't. We are just the same and death is the same for all living things. We can go swiftly, silently and it could happen in an instant.

When the twins are three years old, I meet the Master of the National Maternity Hospital Dublin at a women's talk. 'I remember you,' she says. 'You almost died. It's the best part of my job to see someone like you so healthy now when you came so close to death.'

Nobody knows why I got sepsis. They scratched their heads because it was three whole weeks after the Caesarean. I spent two weeks back on the maternity ward staring at an empty cot. They pumped me full of five different antibiotics. I wish they'd just taken the cot out of the room. I couldn't stop getting sick. I can't look at that neat white baby sheet. Simon's family took the boys during the day. My mother minded the twins without me. She loaded the washing machine again and again. Home at night the boys loaded their loud rage and confusion right back on top of her.

I have a farmer friend whose husband had MND. Through an entire pregnancy she nursed him single-handedly and still ran their farm. The night their daughter was born, she helped him to bed, drove to the hospital and gave birth. The next evening she was back home with their baby. She helped her husband to bed again. True superheroes are so matter-of-fact. They just get on with it and it's no big deal. This woman is mighty. Strength of the land is in her arms.

Home from hospital, I help the nurse get Simon to bed again because there is no carer. The doctor suggests I don't sleep beside him till my scar heals, to avoid more infection, but I can't do that. Our bed is a battleship and it's utter defeat if I leave it. I sleep beside the humming and squelching of pumps and squeaky electrical devices between night feeds. My brain swims in panicky directions. Please, dear brain, just get on with it. Be more matter-of-fact, I beg you. I think of my farmer friend's mighty arms often. She is beautiful and tiny and thin as a whippet. I'd make a lousy farmer. Don't feel sorry for yourself. Don't you dare.

I move through our house feeling slightly perplexed. Where did all these babies come from? As they grow, Pappy the basset hound guards both twins while they play. They sit on him like a hobby horse and pull his sad ears. 'Where is Hunter?' I ask when he's three years old. Busy house and boys don't answer. I find him curled up in a ball in Pappy's basket fast asleep. The dog beside him stares at me gloomily. Hunter my little boy cub has been raised by wolves. His fat cheek rests against fur. Their breaths rise and fall together.

With each birthday my second son Raife begs me for more pets. Many people just don't get it. Why on earth would you say yes? To me it is perfectly obvious. The grim reaper is lurking in my bathroom where the shampoo bottles don't match. This clinical system is out of synch with our souls. What else would we possibly do? This house is our home and our home craves chaos. For some mad reason I will always say yes to more.

Worry

Our eldest, Jack, is a worrier. His mind is a massive island of many inlets. Huge harbours of heavy thoughts moor in hidden crevices. When they get too tied up, BOOM, we get hit. With Jack it could be life or death or just a Lego figure trade gone wrong. Do not underestimate the power of Lego trading. In the heat of the exchange it all seems so right. Soon after, your heart gets ripped by regret, but it's too late. Your favourite Lego figure is in the hands of another, home in some other kid's grubby little pocket. When you're ten this is life and death stuff.

Worry strains his face last thing at night. 'I can't sleep,' he grumbles. 'Just close your eyes and wait,' sighs Arden. 'That's what I do.' We play the relaxing game, an old Jedi mind trick I learned in a faraway yoga class. I whisper words of love and his mind floats off with the moon. His face only ever looks worry-free in the full abandon of boy sleep.

When he was twelve, my eldest brother ran away from boarding school. We were all seated at the kitchen table when a hooded figure shadowed our plates. Worry had him cloaked in darkness and mud. A cartoon misery cloud clearly resided above his head. Chronic asthma made him a bit small for his age. Despite the cloak and cloud, on this day, he looked mighty tall. 'Oh my God!' my mother screamed. The lesson of not hitching a lift had been drilled into him so hard that he walked the entire forty miles home from Dublin. A week later my parents sent him back and he ran away again. He was running for his life. They didn't send him back after that.

Hanging high over rock and sea and train line is the Greystones Cliff Walk. It runs all the way to Bray. Michelle and I like to run with it. Running is great because it requires no skill. Fancy trainers aside, you just put one foot in front of the other. Just keep moving, one step at a time.

Worry is fear that makes your brain wobble. It traps you in a spin cycle and locks you indoors. When I get worried I like to run. Choosing a running partner, it's always best to find a warrior. Michelle is also way fitter than me. I ran with Pappy once but he was too slow. I lost him round a few bends. The sight of his basset hound body, catching up on those short legs, was something to behold.

We drive past the sea every morning on the school run. 'Hello, sea!' shout the five kids. 'Is it good today, Momma?'

asks Sadie. Tide in means a step swim and tide out means a clamber on slippy rocks. Both are good. Too rough is the only bad, meaning no swim at all. 'It's a good day,' I reply. 'Hurray!' she cheers. Sadie is quick to scold me when I'm stressed. Her questions come dressed in finger wags. 'Momma, do you need another swim?' queries her sing-song voice. 'Yes, Sadie, I really do,' is my raw reply.

I grew up in an old house. There was no grand distinguished prettiness. The house was just old and kind of ugly. A former hospital during the Famine, people had died there. Old walls are like sponges. They absorb the damp and dead souls. Then they squeeze them out in concentrated creepiness.

My dad's surgery lay at the end of a long corridor, along with the heating switch. Children were sent there at night to turn off the heating. We all dreaded this well-worn path of doom. Siblings took turns to walk alone with the light of the kitchen on their backs. A walk into darkness lay ahead, past a glass cabinet collection of hideous antique dolls. A quick flick of the heating switch in the cold surgery and you were fucked. Lights out had you lost in perpetual black. Run back towards the light, but the warm kitchen was a lifetime away. It meant running full pelt with darkness rolling over your shoulders. Fear roared in your ears. It was a run for your life.

'Leave the door open a crack!' yells Raife. 'I'm scared of the dark!!'

'Don't be afraid of the dark,' I hush. 'It's just a hug on your eyes to help you sleep.' Also, less soothingly, 'You have no idea how easy you've got it. I mean seriously? We don't even *live* in an old house. Try growing up in a creepy ass house like I did. It was a frickin' horror show every night, hiding under sweaty duvets. There is nothing in here but empty cardboard walls – and out there? Cosy street lights!' He chuckles but my words make no difference. Darkness breathes down your neck as a child and it is primal.

When the moon is out we rush to the front door. My five huddle around me outside. We look up with lunar love to gasp at the stars. The night before Simon returned from ICU, the stars were out in a sparkly dance. Jack wished upon the brightest one for his dad's return. The belief that his wish came true is still stronger than Santa Claus.

There is magic all about, I tell them. Can't you feel it? Jack is encouraged to help his father. Kind nurses show him how the machines work. He runs to place hand warmers under cold fingers. Approval from nurses and family spur him on. He creeps out of the room and I find a worried face cocooned in his bunkbed. 'Jack, it's nice to help,' I say. He nods faithfully. 'You will never ever have to be your dad's nurse, though,' I whisper. His eyes are wide as moons and he grabs hold of me. We hug silently and he won't let go.

*

'Running and swimming?' I sigh. 'Michelle, you have turned me into a total asshole.' We don't belong with any fancy Lycra-wearing, trophy water-bottle, run-with-your-shades-on brigade. Are they actually wearing make-up? This is no show. I still feel compelled to buy a pair of fancy pink trainers though.

Michelle has an uncanny ability to run and talk at the same time. Tragic wives run almost side by side. I am always a few paces behind. 'Keep up, Pappy!' Michelle laughs from up ahead. Don't be fooled by the chat. Michelle and I are running for our lives.

We run to let our feet hit hard earth, to fall and stumble on rocks. We run because it wakes us up to be on a hill high above worry and pain and loneliness. We are sorely alive to the beauty and sadness of this life. Ignoring our souls' hunger is too dangerous a game. We run the legs off our souls to keep them content. Like children cooped up inside for too long on a rainy day, our souls require running feet.

Worried brains will wobble and trick you. My worried brain doesn't want to run the Cliff Walk or swim in the sea. Stay safe, don't bother. A worried brain will have me crouched in the corner, my soul clanking like an empty wine glass.

Up a few steps and running turns worriers into warriors. One foot in front of the other. The Cliff Walk hangs high above the sea. We stare down at the tides that are so change-able. Crashing one day and a still lake the next, tides change, but they are always beautiful. We gaze out at the sea, searching the horizon for love. Our minds cut corners and run tangents. Our legs climb hills and they are free.

We finish our runs by the cove steps and Michelle glances at me with a glint in her eye. This girl is trouble. Suddenly we are peeling off clothes before our run-fuelled bodies cool down. We skip down the steps in our knickers and sports bras. Giggling madly we throw ourselves in. The water never felt colder. Giggles turn quickly to shrieks. Sweaty running gear gets rejected when we climb back out. In the car my toes grip the foot pedals and shaky hands hold the wheel as I drive home barefoot and dripping, swaddled in towels.

'I'm worried that you're just running away,' says a dear worried friend. 'You say it makes you feel better but are you really dealing with your problems? No offence but I don't even *like* sea swimming. It's so tedious and the beach is kind of boring. It's not like it can really fix anything, is it?' I laugh out loud at her honesty. There is no fixing MND. Some things cannot be fixed. I would rather run with magic, thanks.

When I am compelled to jump in the sea, I think of my brother who ran away. He is my chronic asthmatic, heart of a lion, forty-mile hero. Running for your life, you run with gut instinct. Through the rolling of waves, those instincts are rock solid.

Don't worry, Jack, please don't worry. Today I cried for Jack. For his worry about becoming his dad's nurse. For the people who casually championed that seed in his head. For the hug of relief he wrapped around me. Embrace the stars, Jack. Worriers can become warriors. The moon and the stars come gift-wrapped in darkness. Embrace them all. Run with all your heart and everything will be OK.

Lost Things

Lost shoes are a permanent problem in our home. 'It's gone! It's just GONE!' wails Raife, running around the house. He limps into the kitchen with a single secure foot and one sorry-looking exposed sock. My children are wildly dramatic about missing footwear. Shoes are not misplaced. They are gone for ever. Most mornings find us engaging our detective brains in the greatest hunt of all time. The incredible mystery of the missing shoe.

I am sitting in my car in an underground shopping centre, feeling very out of control. I'm not sure what caused this feeling. There are at least ten, which means, minus exaggeration, five reasons why I am having some kind of breakdown. I'm not sure if it is a breakdown, but I can't breathe right, eat right, my hands are numb and waves of nauseating panic ripple like a tide through my day.

On good days, Simon creates treasure hunts on his computer. Our kids love a good mystery. We print off his rhyming clues and giddy nurses hide them around the house. The final prize of books, comics or chocolate bars could be hidden in the garden shed or buried in a flower pot. I draw the line at hiding prizes up the chimney.

This is fun.
This is the place you put your bum.
On the fish.
So make a wish.
Don't do a poo.
And see if you can find the clue.

Write it down, Ruth; tease it out and write it down. I am hoping if I eloquently articulate my breakdown, it will cease to be one. I won't give in to this uncontrollable urge to throw my phone out the window, drive to the Midlands, book into a hotel and hide, sleep, cry under a duvet until someone finds me there and politely asks me to leave. All I can find to write with in this messy car is a blunt fat child's pencil which means that at least I can rub out the words.

We place imaginary Sherlock deerstalkers on our heads each morning in the hunt for lost shoes. 'A prize for whoever finds the shoe!' I yell, in a screaming mother holler because I am lacking an actual referee whistle. Five eager Watsons scramble under beds and lift couch cushions with the prospect of prize jelly babies before school.

Basil, rosemary and chives.
Momma grows these
to make dinners come alive.
Out with the butterflies and birds.
The treasure is in the herbs!

This may seem far-fetched, but parked in the shiny underground car park, I crawled into the back of the car and covered myself in the dog's blanket. I would have slept too, only a coldness was seeping into my bones, particularly at the gap between my jeans and an inadequately warm T-shirt top.

Raife of the lost shoe stands bereft with his hands in the air. It's time to sweeten his soul and quell disaster. 'Let's think,' I soothe. We retrace his rubber-soled steps before they became bedraggled socks. 'It's GONE,' he insists, like a mighty death has occurred.

'Counting up my demons,' sings Chris Martin on the car radio and I couldn't agree more. Write the demons down and they cease to have power. Five reasons for a breakdown stack snuggly one on top of the other. Simon can't move. *That's OK*. Twenty-four hour nurses alternate efficiency, kindness, mess, insanity, privacy theft, bin savagery, toilet hogging, night footsteps, chatty voices and they're EVERYWHERE. *Easy peasy.* The carers join them drinking lots of tea. *Fine.* Five beautiful children love, scream, laugh and plead with me every single day. *Lovely.* A basset hound of increasingly bad attitude growls with a sore skin condition, lives slave to his nose, steals food from tables and snaps when I try and move him. *I can handle it.*

None of these things are causing my breakdown. These things are easy compared to one impossible thing. My dad has cancer and is losing his hair. It's white now and stubbly where once it was dark and full. He is a snow-white fox with bone marrow cancer. If he loses those big eyebrows framing his handsome face, I will die. *This is it.* This is the one thing that has broken me.

I make it out of the car and walk to a bright, busy coffee shop. I sit alone and contemplate lost things. Suddenly the bustle of this place has a swirly, surreal timbre like underwater sounds. I am drowning underwater, swimming breathless with a shoal of colourful fish. Outwardly I am a woman sitting alone mechanically lifting her coffee cup. My face must look a bit freaky, I consider, but nobody glancing has recoiled in horror yet.

Perhaps, I wonder, if the five other reasons weren't stacked so high, I could be a brave daughter in the face of my dad's cancer. I could take it all on and do things. I could speak in a fast voice and walk myself ragged up the solid steps of sickness. I watch my mother do all of this and she is brilliant. I watch her nostalgically like a wise eighty-year-old woman watches the young. Bless 'em.

I did all of this before. I've walked each step already. I am an old woman when I look at my mother. I admire fondly the process she is going through. Where I live now is somewhere outside that process. I miss being that wife. I miss it like breathing right or waking in the morning with the ease of a new day. I sit in my rocking chair, gaze down my bifocals and squint at her with love and envy. I envy her because cancer has a plan of action in a normal land. MND is a medical shoulder-shrug in this batshit crazy town.

The shoe was found today, wedged under the Millennium Falcon. Arden the Victorious holds the shoe aloft. We cheer. The school run is back on track. A triumphant hand stretches out for jelly babies and four more hands follow suit. My mother always had stashes of jellies and treats hidden away for emergencies and our house is no different. If they're not hunting for shoes, the kids are happily plotting how to raid my secret stash.

This is new.
It holds the food.
Momma loves it.
And if she's in the mood.

She might give you a cold treat from here.

It also holds my beer.

So wear your mittens and be bold.

This clue is in the cold.

Is there a point at which humans break? Losing your mind might feel like a child's lost shoe. 'It's just GONE,' I will wail. I've been here before and my breakdown was really the build-up to a good cry. Each time I think, here we go, my sanity is leaving me and what will it feel like? Will I dribble and sit on a hard mattress among white walls? Will I smile at my kids as I float away? Will I walk for miles, barefoot until my feet bleed and will they track me down through credit card transactions?

On bad days Simon sleeps a lot and struggles to connect. We linger at the bedroom door, listening for signs of life. He is trying his best, but not every day is made of rhyming clues. I wonder if Michelle ever feels like this? Some days my man is mostly lost to me. We are left with the architecture and missing furniture. On bad days I hesitate in empty hallways and wonder if we should wake him.

The truth is that ease got lost a long time ago. Ease is like the easily misplaced shoe. I can survive without ease and spend mornings searching for it. I can drink too much coffee, keep busy, alternate cold swims and runs with too much red wine and cheesy nachos. If ease can go astray so efficiently, I wonder, where is my breaking point?

You found me! Well done!
Are you having fun?
The next clue is not at all scary,
it's in the bed of one of the fat fairies!

This could be the greatest detective mystery of all time. What happens if the second shoe is sanity and it gets stolen too? What then? It's bloody lucky that shoes never seem to go missing in pairs. Dear God, give this woman a jelly baby. Are we there yet? Here we go. I leave my empty coffee cup on the counter and head to the newsagent's to buy a pen.

Wolf or Panda

'Would you rather be poor and everyone loves you, or really rich and everybody hates you?' My boys are full of critical questions. They must be considered carefully and answered instantly. 'Just answer the question, Momma, quick!'

'Would you rather die by a great white shark or live like a vampire?'

'Dying by a shark would be better because it's quick,' reasons Arden sagely. The others grumble their agreement. 'What do you think, Momma?'

'What, huh?' I falter, spinning three steaming pots on the stovetop simultaneously.

'Which would you rather be, Momma, a wolf or a panda?' demands Raife. 'Pick one!' I think of a large veggie panda chewing on bamboo all day. 'Oh a panda, definitely,' I reply.

'Well, Momma?' berates Raife with a tongue click, 'the truth is that being a panda is actually kind of stressful. If a mother panda has more than one baby she has to choose one and leave the other little pink babies to die. Then the father panda leaves every time and she has do everything by herself.'

'Jesus,' I mutter, 'and I just thought pandas were cute hippies.'

'Wolves, though,' continues Raife, 'will only hurt you if they're threatened. When a wolf family grows and grows they never break apart, they stay together for ever and ever till they're dead'.

'You got all this from kids' *National Geographic*?' I marvel. 'Wow, that's deep stuff'.

'I told you, I have a golden brain,' he shrugs, snatching the sauce spoon for a lick.

Sea swimming does wonders for your inhibitions. For the first few weeks I cowered self-consciously on the cove steps. My baby-battered body felt exposed. These days we shed clothes like discarded sweet wrappers. The packaging is incidental. We climb out of the water like mermaid goddesses. Cold water gives us new skin.

Simon is shooting his film, *My Name is Emily*. I look at him proudly. He inhabits a magical state of mind. No longer the man in the bed, he is the first film director with MND to ever make a feature film using an eye gaze computer. He draws up deep resources and burns the brightest. Producers carefully construct the schedule around half-days for him, just in case. Nobody could have anticipated the fire in him. He is on set every day from dawn till dusk.

I sneak a look at Raife's magazine. Wolves look like loners and yet they are loyal to the death. One of their greatest strengths is strong emotional attachments to others. Raife, I've changed my mind. My eyes are increasingly intense and wolflike. I crave meat and my own company. I am living a wolf's life. Wolves cannot be domesticated. My messy house can vouch for that. MND has cultivated a certain wolfishness. I don't want to be a stressed-out panda, feeling abandoned, chewing bamboo all day. Forget endangered and tragic, I won't dangle near extinction. Little Red Riding Hood was such a little idiot. Don't mess with me. I want to be a wolf.

Simon is fully charged and lovesick at work. He lives in that creative place many of us crave. Commitment issues prevent most of us from lingering there long enough. Fear and self-consciousness lock us out. Simon's focus is unshakeable. Find a way in and you are dragged towards this place and nowhere else. It pulls you closer to yourself and the reason you exist at all. He is off making a movie and I am so damn happy for him. I look at his empty bed and am inspired to use this time constructively. I decide to get naked as often as possible.

'In the nip! We're in the nip!' my children shout as bare bottoms jiggle in the hallway. I envy them because I detest locked doors. Demure disrobing is demanded of me in my very public house. Simon and nurses leave for the film set every morning in a hub of activity. The house now settles into different sounds. Bathroom doors stay open. Oh, the luxury of a hot shower with doors thrown wide and a knickers & bra trail mapping the floor. I join the naked pack running up and down the hall. 'Momma's in the nip too!' they squeal. Friends call on the phone and they know. 'You're naked, aren't you?' they sigh. 'Oh yes,' I beam. We steer clear of Skype and Facetime.

Vans, tents and cables collect at Greystones South Beach on a soft Irish morning. It's one of those wonky days when the rain seems to fall skywards. Drizzle rises under umbrellas and soaks you from the ground up. Simon is shooting his film all around Wicklow and we often play Spot the Catering Van in between school runs. Today is a special day. Simon sits in his director's tent, wrapped up and full of intent, glaring hungrily at the camera monitor. One hundred extras shuffle around the beach in bathrobes, nervously sipping hot soup. Concealed by misty rain clouds, there's still no hiding that this is a public beach.

Michelle tells us stories about past swims with Galen. The Forty Foot is a popular swimming spot in Dublin. One man in his sixties used to star-jump naked before diving in. Understandably, this image has stayed with Michelle. He was very hairy, she says. He would star-jump for a good ten minutes.

Brief silence descends on Ladies' Cove as we all take room to contemplate the idea of this man properly.

Our nurse, Marian, gives me a strange-looking lamp as a present. It is a large clump of rock with a light inside. 'It's a salt lamp,' she explains. 'They absorb all the bad energy in your house.' The salt rock glows bright orange when the light turns on. It has a cosy hearth glow. Bad energy is a baffling mystery, but it's worth a try. Orange is the colour of home and I love it.

The wind whispers tales of sweet abandon at the cove. We all listen. An old lady in flowing robes gently deposits an ancient ghetto blaster on the stones. Tin-can tribal music warbles across the rocks. She proceeds to dance around it, arms circling the air in a crazy old lady dance. The children prowl closer. 'She doesn't even *see* us!' they chuckle. 'She's mad as a brush,' I mutter. I ponder the freedom of hairy naked man and the dancing lady. I could star-jump stark naked in my eighties, boobs and wobbly bits bouncing wildly, happy in my own skin, hoping I don't have a bad hip. Could I go there? Never say never.

There are red faces one day as my father-in-law forgets Simon is out on the film set. He uses his key to let himself in. I have just left the shower, towelless and singing loudly. Songs turn to screams and the slap of wet, mortified retreating foot-steps. After that, he always knocks first.

*

On the *My Name Is Emily* film shoot, exhibitionists, fellow MND sufferers, fundraisers, local friends and random lunatics have all turned out at South Beach to support Simon. They line up facing the sea and remove their robes. Laughter ripples through the air as men and women, of every shape and size, huddle together bollock naked. Actor Michael Smiley is out front. He's in the nip with a glint in his eye. A rubber codpiece preserves some modesty. The cameras roll and he yells to the crowd, 'This is who we are! COME ON!' His bare bum races towards the water and a blur of one hundred naked bottoms follows. A tribal roar rises up. Every film should have one massive nude sea shot. Safe on the prom-enade in raingear, we watch and get goosebumps. It's a bit like a beach-themed *Braveheart*.

The cameras roll for just one take and I struggle to take it all in. Like most amazing sights it is unreal and dreamlike. We avert our eyes respectfully, as the naked extras return up the beach. Full frontals swing ferociously as legs clamber back up the sand. Running on dry sand never looked so ungainly. The boys' tennis coach, a proper lady in her sixties, and a friendly mum from the school gates, both greet me glowingly, once back in their bathrobes. 'Would Jack like to come on a playdate tomorrow?' asks the mum politely. The world has gone wonderfully mental I think as I nod yes. I am utterly speechless. Laughing crying tears gather in my eyes. The power of this lot hums louder than the catering generators.

They are all high as kites. One hundred naked people on Greystones beach is one of the most beautiful things I have ever seen.

Marian phones me on one of her nights off. Her voice is filled with urgency. 'It's a full moon, Ruth,' she says briskly. 'Now listen carefully. The salt lamp I gave you. Get it. You need to wrap the plug in clingfilm and then put it outside. I'm putting mine on the grass to keep it grounded, but your table outside will do fine.' I shush the kids with an arm wave. 'Did you hear all of that?' she demands.

'Salt lamp, clingfilm, table outside,' I repeat. 'Dare I ask why?'

'The salt lamp is absorbing all the bad energy in your house. Leaving it overnight under the full moon empties it out again.'

'I'd say it's pretty full, all right,' I grin. Marian's laugh is like a bell. 'I know you think I'm mad, but in pagan times people used to lie naked under the full moon to absorb its energy. The Harvest Moon especially.'

'Marian, you are completely nuts and I love you. I'll do it, but only if we make a deal. Let's lie naked under the next Harvest Moon, because *that* sounds like a fun night.'

'You could *swim* naked under the Harvest Moon,' giggles Marian: 'that sounds more your type of night.'

*

I carefully clingfilm my salt lamp and leave it outside. The moon is massive and cut like a dish. I smile and moongaze for some sweet moments. A naked full moon swim. What a wonderful idea. I want to tell my Tragic Wives, Michelle and Aifric. Let's moon swim to empty out our souls.

Endangered lives have a stressed-out panda shape. Full moon swims fall violently out of my head one carelessly horrible day. I get a call from the hospital about a car accident. Marian has crashed and she is broken.

Sea glass

We live our lives in fragments and that's just the way it is. Clocks circling time have little meaning for me. From days and months to moments, fragments of time swing solely between good and bad. I never dare presume, beyond a hunch, what is coming next.

Sadie is standing in front of our wedding photograph, sobbing her little heart out. 'Why didn't I go to the wedding?' she weeps. 'Why can't Dadda talk or walk? Is he sick? Is Dadda OK? Will he stay with us for ever?' Oh no and here we go, screams my brain. I had wondered if this day would come. 'Why can't he go back to the old Dadda who walked and talked? Was that just the olden days?' I grab her tiny body in a bear hug. Whispering into wet cheeks, I wish I was more prepared. Words curdle to cheesiness in such moments. 'He's still the same Dadda in his heart and he loves you so much,' I offer. 'Why can't the old Dadda come OUT of his heart? she demands, crushing my cartoon words. Toddler logic easily decimates Disney platitudes.

I was a bridesmaid at a friend's wedding. At the hen party, we spent happy hours in a pottery cafe. I painted a plate for Simon inspired by my favourite Winnie-the-Pooh quote. Piglet sits quivering on a windy day. '*"Supposing a tree fell down, Pooh, when we were underneath it?" "Supposing it didn't," said Pooh after careful thought.*' Pooh and Piglet hold hands in silhouette on my plate, surrounded by swirly orange and yellow blobs. The words 'Supposing it didn't' circle their feet. That plate has stayed with us from house to house and now stands guard over the boys' bunk beds.

Marian has crashed her car and is in the emergency room. When I get the call I go numb. My brain gets bossy and tells me to get up and go to her because I cannot just sit at home. I frantically think of things Marian likes. Nice books get grabbed from our bookshelves and I race to Tesco for a bag of hot chicken wings. Marian loves spicy chicken wings.

'I wish he was the Dadda in the olden days. He just turned into a different Dadda because it wasn't the olden days any more,' Sadie reasons. 'How long is it gonna be till the olden days again?' I carry my beautiful girl to bed, stroking her hair. 'It's OK to feel sad, everyone gets sad sometimes. I will always love you, Sadie,' I croon into her curls. 'Everyone loves me in this town,' she yawns, eyes heavy on her pillow. 'Yes, Sadie, everyone in this town loves you,' I chuckle. 'I don't want to grow up because my pyjamas are still only tiny,' she mumbles, falling into that deep sleep of the emotionally spent. Tears still cling to her lashes. Hunter snores beside her, dreaming of dogs.

The emergency room is a horrible hellish place and I know it so well. Moans and shouts mix with the constant scrape of cubicle curtains that open and close. Overworked hospital staff march around beds. They look more like stressed-out plumbers, frantically patching up leaks. This is no hospital, we are in Purgatory, a waiting place between worlds. I have lost days in here with Simon. Time has no meaning in this brightly lit land. There are no windows. Large headaches loom under long fluorescent strip lights.

I snake expertly through beds, searching for Marian. There is sadness in the knowledge that I can navigate these floors with such ease. So many nurses and staff send a nod my way because they know me. A good handful have been through my home. Knickers hanging on my kitchen clothes horse are known to them by colour. They could probably pinpoint the exact patterns on all my pyjamas.

I fall upon her family standing startled around a bed. This is a body I don't recognise. Marian's face is bloated and bruised. Her small frame is twisted around a back brace and she is groaning in agony. 'I brought chicken wings,' I falter, holding them aloft like a fool. The idea that Marian could read books or eat chicken wings right now is completely insane. Her husband takes the chicken politely. 'They're still a bit warm,' I add hopefully. His smile conveys thanks, like all he's ever wanted is this rapidly cooling bag of congealed wings. In that moment, meeting him for the first time, I know he is a kind man. I ramble nonsense, deposit my reading material and leave, feeling utterly useless. This is how our friends felt when Simon got sick, I realise, running from the place. God, it feels totally shit.

After three weeks in Purgatory, Marian is sent home with a fractured vertebra. I visit her house in Wicklow and this time I bring cake. The door is opened by a broken woman who can barely walk. I am horrified that she even answered the door. She shuffles back to the kitchen and insists on making tea. Her hands can't even lift the kettle. Black pools of pain are clouding her eyes. All of her lightness is gone. She forces a smile that tells me this angel is now living in Hell.

'Oh, Ruth, it was so violent.' She shivers, talking about the accident. She covers her eyes with both hands, like a frightened child. A car came out from a slip road too fast and she swerved to avoid it. Hitting the motorway middle barrier, her car flipped three times. She had unclicked her seat belt moments earlier to reach for something and got thrown from the car window like a rag. Her body was left broken on the road.

Marian's car is like Mary Poppins's carpet bag. From toilet rolls to spare teabags, light bulbs, motion-sensor bathroom lights and boxes of chocolate Weetos, Marian can fetch any household shortage straight from her car. Coat stands and tassled lamps wouldn't surprise me either. All of these things got thrown on to the road with her, along with the pretty pink cardigan she was knitting for Sadie. 'You must have blacked out,' I pleaded. No, she was awake the entire time. She lay on the road and one of her first thoughts was, who will mind Simon now? When the ambulance arrived she yelled at them to get Sadie's knitting off the road.

'I'm not going anywhere,' Marian promised me once. My eyes tear up at the memory. Marian may never be fit to nurse again. Books and newspapers are piled on her precious piano in the sitting room, because she can no longer play. 'I'm not going anywhere' I want to promise back, but I can't find the words. Fractured lives with nurses and ventilators mean I can never promise anything. Tomorrow doesn't exist yet and I won't be held by promises.

I go home to my children who are beating the crap out of each other. 'Something bad happened,' says Arden ominously. We go to the bedroom. Three boys stand in collective culpable silence. My Winnie-the-Pooh plate lies shattered in pieces. A stray shoe hit and smashed it to the floor. The plate is broken and suddenly I just break along with it. I kneel on the floor, spilling tears with crumbling delft. Why am I crying? It's only a thing, I scold myself. Eyes still gushing, I try to glue the pieces, but my vision is blurry. Swirly blobs of yellow and orange are too cracked. I can't glue them back properly. Everything breaks. I feel so damaged, glued, chipped and not the same. *'Supposing it didn't'*? Oh shut up, Pooh Bear – go run off with Disney. It bloody well just did and there's no supposing. I wearily hang the wonky plate back up again. It clings precariously to the wall but doesn't fall.

We go to the cove and the children run. Arden has been silent since the plate incident. Cross words were exchanged. I sit gloomily on a rock and look out to sea. The water looks harsh and formidable. I shiver and don't feel like swimming. New nurses will come and change the shape of our home again. I miss Marian so much. Nobody could understand. I stare at impossible big waves and brush away tears so the kids can't see. Even those closest to us have their own lives. They have hobbies and trips to escape to, partners who share tasks, a daily routine that doesn't include us. I crave those escapes. Our routine is us and we are exhausting to live with.

Arden walks alone near the water's edge. He is my hardy beachcomber boy with a cowboy heart. All good cowboys like to stand solo, just a few steps out of reach. Some fragments still hold joy. I think of Simon's magic pocket on his pyjamas. We fill it with treats for little hands to find. Five in the bed with him watch *Britain's Got Talent*, laughing at performing dogs and daring tricks. These fragments sit like stones in my pocket. Today's pain has a shape too solid.

I feel sadness on a deep level, deeper than skin and veins and death. Clock hands circling time are overwhelming and endless. The sea looks so rough it might hurt, so I breathe in the salt air and stare at the rocks. Arden strolls up behind me. He places something in my hand without speaking. I look down in surprise. Three beautiful bits of sea glass gleam in my palm. He grins a cheeky grin. 'Does this mean we're friends again?' I hiccup, openly crying now. 'Yes!' he shouts into the wind, already walking away.

I smile as my soul soars out to sea. A cowboy will always break your heart. With cowboys you are at least guaranteed a good clean break. My heart is in sea-glass pieces and I am saved. I hold on to my new fragments that sparkle like diamonds.

Christmas

When you live with MND, milestones become difficult. We wander shell-shocked along uneven roads. Milestones at regular intervals bring you out in full body sweats. Birthdays and Christmas are such heavy rocks. They can't be ignored and feel too cumbersome to carry.

We've spent most of our MND years struggling with Christmas. Coming from two equally Christmas-obsessed families, Simon and I harboured Yuletide yearnings all year round. From the first, we divvied up holiday time like junkies.

It is probably way cooler to dismiss Christmas as an existential distraction. Cynics cry that Christmas is just one more colourful way to avoid the fact that we're all going to die. Drown them out with a Wham! tune, will you? Bring out the cherished Christmas Number Ones compilation. We're too distracted in our Christmas jumpers, kissing under mistletoe, to notice.

I was always a Christmas fool. I believe in magic. I believed in Santa until my mother took me aside at a shocking age. I was stubborn, even after my brothers showed me secret presents. I still squint to make sure the lights are evenly distributed on the tree and get lost in a shaft of sparkly tinsel.

Birthdays are approached like battlegrounds. For Simon's birthday we dice with different designs. Dice can often leave you at a loss so just roll with it. For the man who can't eat, one year we make a playdough cake. The twins try and eat it for him. What do you buy the man who cannot move, taste or smell? Coffee, whiskey and DVDs, please. If we're really stumped, there's always socks.

Christmas became difficult. Families felt awkward eating around tables. Their good hearts tried to keep everything the same. Meals were subtly restructured with buffets, but our faces were strained. Seeing how different we were from our siblings' laughing family units hurt the most. I marvelled at the ease of other couples. There even seemed to be joy in their arguments.

For Simon's 40th in September, I have to think bigger. I want to rock his world. Aifric puts me in touch with an artist friend of her sister. I paint the wall outside our bedroom window white, muttering about grey depressing brick. My idea is to paint a mural so the man in the bed has a magical view. Our new artist friend Mick has more mind-blowing ideas. He gathers pieces from fellow artists all around Dublin to be hung on the wall in rotation, so that Simon's view will constantly change.

After silently munching croissants in the kitchen, a crowd gathers at the bedroom door. We pull back the curtains to reveal Mick's beautiful wood sculpture depicting the two main characters from Simon's film. A procession of sparkler-holding children march by the window, waving and smiling. There are several technical glitches with sound as Hunter keeps pressing the CD buttons. Glitches are to be expected when you work with children.

Art is on the move, outside the window, swift and fast, passed by Aifric, with baby on hip, to Simon's brother-in-law, who straightens each piece. I read out the name of each artist to lots of oohing and aahing. Aifric's husband Phil has made a large portrait of our five children sitting on grass. They point up to a magical cloud castle in the sky. This one has the birthday boy in tears.

It is our biggest birthday success, and it's all over in ten minutes. Simon leaves with his nurses for the film set because he is no longer the man in the bed. The film director doesn't need a new view. He's making his own.

'ISN'T THERE ANYONE WHO KNOWS WHAT CHRISTMAS IS ALL ABOUT?'

So roared Charlie Brown in his 1960s Christmas movie. His buddy Linus, with the blanket, gave a speech about baby

Jesus and the King of Kings. But it wasn't the answer I was looking for. I love the way Charlie shouts this in a moment of pure anguish. I never understood anguish at Christmas until our cuddly Christmas blanket got pulled away. Anguish is the draught that leaves you cold and shivery.

These days Christmas presents are badly wrapped. We have a nurse roster ripped full of holes. There is far too much Sellotape. Holiday nurses arrive who don't know Simon. Often they lack a certain luminance, like lost Christmas ghosts. They drift between jobs for the season and sleep in lonely agency hostels. It might be unkind to say that many of them are total weirdos.

We have room-for-rent smiles on our faces as the Christmas nurses wander in. Some are bad nurses you want to bat back out the door. Nurse roster? There is no nurse roster. January looks like Swiss cheese. I'd be better off standing on street corners. HEY! You've got a nice face! Come with me and join our family!

This living situation hurts. But isn't that just so boring? Pain is so boring now. I come home and a new carer has pulled out my entire wardrobe and laid it on the bed to be tidied. I am a messy girl. She pulls my things apart and puts them back together better, neater, lovelier. Her smile is so kindly. I am horrified, violated and then laughing, because it's absurd. This is so absurd I can't even get offended. Also, it is so much tidier.

*

With Simon's birthdays, I am armed for battle. With my own, I run for cover. People keep buying me plants. My heart plummets in the knowledge that without Marian, these plants are doomed to die. Simon is assisted by family in buying and wrapping my presents. Written by another hand and wrapped so neatly, they bring me no joy. His family means well, but this hurts. I shove my heart into my boots and pull the laces up tight. If this is the way presents have to be, I would rather have none. Perhaps that is childish, but it is too large a reminder of all my husband cannot do. I don't want presents passed through many hands. I don't want anything. I'm no martyr, I am actually high maintenance because all I want is love.

We should have turned into some kind of resentful, warped Grinch monster of anarchy, hating Christmas shitness. Yet somehow, this time of year still gets me. I'm not even religious. I still believe in magic. I don't know how after everything that has happened to us. At the annual school carol service I wonder if it's all that collective singing togetherness.

Christmas time tickles me into comas of confusion with sick kids, no nurses and a blur of Christmas adverts on the radio that make me want to smash something. Like many worries, the prospect of Christmas looms larger than the reality.

When Christmas Day finally hits, it is so busy. We get

Simon to his family in one piece. The boys and I build a train table for Hunter that fills up our entire hall. Jack, Raife and Arden sport fake moustaches and laser guns from their Santa stockings. They happily stalk each other around the house. Every time I turn around Raife has new lip fluff of different colour and shape.

Sadie runs down the hall shouting, 'THIS IS THE BEST CHRISTMAS EVER!!!' I laugh knowing that nothing I did really deserved that. Her words come purely from her own enthusiasm. She could have a zombie-flesh-eating catatonic mother and she would still be shouting it.

During the holidays, I get into a Christmas sea so cold my hands shake for an hour afterwards. Raife and I go to the shops. He has to use my card to pay for stuff because hand tremors inhibit my key punches. Quaking crazy fists can't even hold the card. We laugh like proper turn-your-stomach-inside-out kids. The deadpan guy behind the counter looks at us, slightly baffled. 'Are you cold or something?' he asks. Maybe it's my blue lips.

Some things never change. My favourite part of Christmas has always been that dregs of the day moment when the shine wears off. Families fuelled by alcohol fall back into the roles and stereotypes they carry for life. I am immersed in the same sibling fights. The same unspoken resentments linger. Messy midnight charades end in age-old arguments and childish huffs.

Sleigh bells ring to the quiet revelation that the perfect lives of our siblings are not always so happy. Couples stress and snap at each other. Are you listening? I love all these people to my very bones. Living in this vortex of no nurses and endless days in pyjamas, I think that leading a vaguely unhappy, normal, stressed and snappy life might be nice to try some time, just for a few weeks. Then I find a really good murder mystery book to dive into and I stop thinking so much altogether.

When my birthday comes around, Phil and Aifric visit after Simon has returned to bed. Phil is always named first because, phonetically, they must avoid becoming 'African Phil'. We drink wine until Phil, ever the gentleman, bows out gracefully to facilitate girlie chats. By candlelight and red wine, we reminisce in a way unique to those who've been friends since the age of three. There is an ease of shared space and a deep appreciation of each other's company. We laugh and cry and whisper as only girls can.

It is 5 a.m. when Aifric finally shuffles out the door. 'You were always so cool and aloof in school,' she declares. 'Like you didn't need anyone. As a friend that made you so attractive.' Perhaps I really am a wolf, I marvel. Aloofness back then merely masked a girl who was painfully shy. The birthday martyr just got all the love she could need. I am drunk. Thank God for my Wishing-Well Friend.

*

Another Christmas is over as tree baubles hang heavy and branches begin to sag. The hoover sucks up the fallen needles with a satisfying noisy finality. The weight of another milestone has lifted. Sadie storms into the kitchen and roars cross-eyed with tiredness, 'GIVE ME SOMETHING TO EAT OR CHRISTMAS IS RUINED!' Oh fickle-hearted maiden. I'm laughing more than the Best Christmas Ever.

Bed

'I think I might be in love', says Raife, matter-of-factly. 'A girl in school keeps bumping into me.'

'Does it feel like your heart falls into your stomach when you look at her?' asks Jack quietly.

'YES!' shouts Raife. 'But how did YOU know that, Jack?'

'Oh there was a girl in France by the pool,' sighs Jack. 'I never talked to her, I just looked at her from far away.'

Years before Simon and I kissed, I fell asleep at a student party. My drunken body crashed out on the nearest empty bed. I woke in the morning with a fright. A man's face was facing mine and it wasn't my boyfriend's. Our noses were nearly touching. Simon had crawled into the space between me and the wall, to sleep beside me during the night. He would later claim drunken innocence. I fled before he woke up because I had no choice. My heart was falling into my stomach repeatedly. His body had deliberately bumped into mine. That handsome face lingered with me for weeks.

Wolves make a bond for life. We can no longer hold each other and wrap limbs together. When machinery, air mattresses and tubes distort distances between you, how do you hold on to your wolf bond? I wish in urgent whispers for an answer.

When we moved back to Greystones, our marital bed became a hospital contraption. It had multiple tilts and reclining functions. We are mid-thirties eighty-year-olds with a bed built for easy TV watching. Sit up. Lie back. Raise your legs. For the first month our mattresses reeked like a plastic ashtray. The previous occupant had been a big smoker. He died and left a scent. Simon's side of the bed soon needed his own motorised air mattress. In the most romantic of gestures, he bought me a fancy pocket-sprung double-layered single for my side, complete with a quilted mattress protector. Farewell to cold slippery foam. I no longer slept on Dead Man's smoke stench.

I lie on my well-padded mattress at a moderate tilt with restless pulsing limbs. My feet feel oversized and swollen. Motors hum like machine guns all around me. Television sounds seep into my dreams. This bedroom is a sensory assault of sound, light and equipment. I am locked in a half-dream. Benedict the night nurse is slapping cream on Simon repeatedly and I can smell it. He massages limbs and I am engaged in a small earthquake.

I cover my face with the duvet and then my brain does an odd thing. It starts chanting the Lord's Prayer in a frantic holy loop. Funny brain, why do you resort to this mantra? As a little girl I found solace kneeling before home-made Catholic altars. I dressed them with frilly tablecloths, statues and flower-filled egg cups of bluebells and snowdrops. I was so good. Maybe I still yearn to be good. It's more likely I'm just desperate.

I take to sitting in cars again. Hunter sleeps in his car seat holding a naked plastic baby. Sadie is snoring. I wish I could sleep and wake up renewed, but I never do. I would love to sleep for a month, be on my own for a month, leave and live in isolation to think and drink tea, hear the clock tick, and rest my limbs on a quiet bed. All I have are these bleary warm moments in cars and it's never enough to feel restored.

When my mother was a girl she fell asleep on a picnic blanket in a grassy field. She woke with a persistent pain in her ear. The pain was dull at first. It grew in intensity until she could bear it no more. Her father finally took some tweezers to her ear and pulled out a big fat earwig. This monstrous thing had nestled into warm waxy crevices and locked pincers around her inner ear.

'Tell us the earwig story!' we would beg my mother as kids. 'Please!' It was by far our favourite tale. Without exception, as adults we are all now morbidly terrified of earwigs, pincer tails and all. It's the kind of fear that makes the most rational eyes water with horror.

Annagassan beach in Co. Louth is vast and flat. When the tide is out, miles of soft sand make it the perfect terrain for galloping horses. As a child I visit with a friend whose mother keeps horses. She leaves us playing in puddles while she gallops wildly towards a distant line of blue sea.

Our boots begin to sink until suddenly we are engulfed in quicksand. Laughing and whooping we realise that we are permanently stuck. This is the attack of the dreaded sand monster. We are daredevils locked in a great adventure. Still laughing, our eyes frantically search the horizon for that horse silhouette.

We exist in a pocket of time that feels endless. What if she doesn't come back? How long can we last? Wellies are sucked under and the sand rises up to our knees. Our hands sink up to our elbows as we fall forward. The laughing stops. We fall silent.

Our saviour returns on horseback. She finds two half-sunken little girls with legs boasting ever-increasing splits. We are slumped forward and soaked to the skin. The mother pulls us out like popped corks. Shivering in our knickers, we huddle under a blanket in the back seat of her car, giggling all the way home.

I was trained in radio production to have alert ears. My

ears and soul are savagely sensitive to music. If a song doesn't suit my mood, I will leave the room in a panic. Perhaps that is why the whirring, squelching and farting of electrical equipment is so hurtful to me. I am also particularly stubborn. When my feet are sinking in sand, I tend to stand stoical. This time I know there is no hope of a horse on the horizon. That makes it so much harder to be brave.

Our marital bed is damaging my soul. It wasn't immediately obvious that it was doing so. Hurt crept into the warm crevices of my ear like a nasty earwig. Only when it dug deep did I feel the pinch. It's a dull ache that grows and grows until one day it is monstrous. I am exhausted. After six years, the ear pinching is unbearable. I make the impossible decision to leave our bed.

For months, I wander the house at night. I pass out on couches and crawl in beside kids like some kind of bed gypsy. There is no solace in the frantic dreams that seem intent on tormenting me. I wake on the hour, two, three, four a.m. At 5 a.m. I give up and shuffle around the house like a monk. *The darkest hour is just before dawn.* I make tea and stare at walls. I see the sun come up and watch it slowly paint the sky.

I don't know how to be this person who doesn't love her bed. I used to tell my husband his imagination would always save him. Now my own dreams torture and prod me all night. I miss my daydreams and the solace of sleep. I miss man skin and wolf bonds and shared beds without alternating pressure functions.

Wolves stay together until they're dead, but what if the death is a really slow one? We are left dangling, daring to hope, not to hope. A slow living death of many plateaus, false alarms and subtle dwindling.

If I was a mermaid, I would send a lonely song out to sea. A single tragic note wailing on the winds. I would hold that note until my breath was gone. Everything I took for granted about myself – all my strengths – seems to have left me. They hightailed it out of a noisy hospital bed that now closely resembles a leaking boat.

I am back to staring at fantastical shapes and faces. They leap out from the wooden slats above my head. I have claimed the spare bottom bunk in the boys' bedroom as my own, with a well-placed teddy and owl cushion. The boys are giddy with excitement. 'We like having you here, Momma,' they giggle with camping adventure delight. I fall asleep to the sweet lullaby of warm, rapid boy-breaths.

My ears are at peace but my head is too busy for sleep. I did my very best, but a deep bond has been broken. Simon sleeps alone with a baby monitor and a nurse listening in. He has 20-minute checks. I love him. But now I just look at him from far away. The silence is deafening. My heart falls into my stomach repeatedly. Our marital bed is gone. I sleep fitfully and wake each morning with a gasp.

Murder

Sadie is skipping around Simon's bed singing in an operatic roar. 'Momma, I don't *want* a big giant Dadda. I just want a tiny Dadda. A Dadda like this one.' This child has no fear of new nurses. She scrambles into every nest, a brazen cuckoo looking for cuddles. Finding a knee to sit on, she smiles sweetly. 'Can I play with your phone?' she demands with her prettiest wide-eyed blink. There may be many knees and phones but there is only one Dadda.

I have thought about murdering my husband. I get these lustful feelings, murderous in the most mysterious way. I don't think a mother could ever feel like this. I think only a wife would. I used to consume Agatha Christie books as a child. Wives would kill their husbands casually with poison and pointed lack of passion, just for money or titles or a house or some land. It was all quite clinical. Nothing like the frenzied feeling of seeing your beloved in anguish. This is primal raw

passion that screams STOP IT! THIS HAS TO END NOW!
It is the chaos of pure wifely love.

Organising the art show for Simon's birthday, I want to
get his window view exactly right. While he is out on the film
set, I lie on his bed to figure out which part of the wall he can
see best. Lying on his noisy air mattress I instinctively decide
to stay still and see how long I can last. Alternating pressure
pockets ripple underneath me and churn my stomach to
seasickness. Thirty seconds in and the urge to move my head
is a loud scream. My eyeballs strain left and right to such a
limited range. Less than a minute passes before I leap from
the bed. I can never fully comprehend his view because it
would break me.

I've accepted these lustful, murderous feelings as completely natural. They make me proud because I could never
actually kill my husband. His suffering is great but he has no
desire to die. There is no guilt. The murderous thoughts only
mean I truly love him. A wife could not claim her beloved
without also claiming a desire to end this much suffering.
There are moments when tears flood his face into a frozen
grimace and his eyes are wild and wretched with agony. When
empathy pulls you into his unscuffed shoes for a mere five
seconds, have a taste of concentrated terror. Even a heart of
stone would be moved to murder, at least for a moment.

Every time love takes me here, I am pulled up short by

our children. They dote on him. They seek him out and put their hands on him. His face glows like a Christmas lantern. His eyes gleam and although there is so little movement left, they shine enough that you know he is at peace. His eyes are set in a different shape. Sadie pats his face, Hunter grins at him. Jack burrows for cuddles, Raife talks his talk and Arden leans nearby in true cowboy style.

Michelle and I are running one day when she doubles over and stops. 'I'm fine, I'll be fine,' she mutters, but she is bleeding. We make it to her house and I leave her reluctantly. 'Go home, Ruth,' she insists, 'my sister will be here any minute.' I have to go home to wash the dog and collect the kids and get the dinner and I should never ever have left Michelle. Her sister arrives to find her collapsed on the bedroom floor. In hospital they diagnose a gastric disorder and put her on a massive dose of steroids. When a mighty warrior falls, we all falter. We can only wait to ask her what the hell we are supposed to do next.

The dog got sick and it gets too much. Pappy, our beloved basset hound, has turned into an asshole, I tell my husband. A chronic skin condition had made him a grumpy bastard for quite some time. He ate something odd in the garden and slumped into a half coma. The vet tried to put him on a drip and he attacked her. 'The next 24 hours will be critical,' warns the vet. 'He has terrible deep veins.' They can't get the drip in. I stare at the dog in wonder. My own veins sit plump and fat on scrawny arms, but Simon's veins are notorious. 'He has terrible deep veins,' say the doctors as they pincushion him at each hospital visit. Oh, God help me. The dog and Simon are united in illness and bad veins.

I pace the floors waiting for word of Pappy's fate. Suddenly I am so angry at the two of them. How dare they both get so sick? Perhaps we need a death. A release from all this pain. A resting place for it. If death is coming, so be it. Better that the dog gets his. Pappy just might be the sacrifice we need. We can sell his canine soul for our own sanctuary. I am ready.

I am not ready. Pappy survives and I take him home in utter relief. My tough talk is total nonsense. I'm no more ready for death than Simon. Pappy's skin continues to worsen. I am bathing him more than the children. At least they don't try and bite me. He growls and snarls at everyone. I barricade myself with couch cushions just to get him out the back door. He lunges at me baring pointy teeth and red gums. I am properly afraid with tears in my eyes. He is a big dog and very strong. One day he bites Arden's best friend's hand and breaks the skin. I am petrified and tell Simon we need to take him back to the vet.

I visit Michelle who is run down but not broken. She is taking her steroids and is resolved to follow a raw food regime to get herself back on track. The warrior doesn't get tragic. There is fire in her eyes. 'We'll run again soon,' she growls at me. Michelle may be a mad raw-food hippie, but she has no doubt. Maybe we're all deluded but I know for sure we will run.

Familiar with Pappy from previous visits, the vet doesn't feign surprise. Pappy greets her by attacking both her and the assistant. He nearly bloody savages them. Maybe he knows what is coming. She says that bassets can go this way and when they do, they only get worse. People can learn to live around them and not piss them off but in a house of five children, that would be impossible. He couldn't be rehomed with his untreatable skin and aggressive streak.

Mother bear kicks in and I know I cannot bring Pappy home. The vet has confirmed all my worst fears. Someone will get hurt. I am not brave enough to go home and bring him back here again. I need her to guide me through this horrible process. I sit and hold him while she puts him to sleep. It is the worst thing I have ever done, but I cannot let him back among our children. Simon had suggested his mum might take him. I won't offload a problem dog on a good lady I love, who is already carrying so much. I don't want anyone to live with the guilt of this decision but me. I have failed the dog and I am the one who will carry it.

I whisper into his warm fur as the big blue syringe begins to take effect. His breathing gets slower. The vet quietly leaves the room. I weep over him and stroke him as I whimper, 'Sorry, sorry, Pappy . . . I'm so sorry I called you an asshole.' There is no forgiving this, but I beg the dog anyway as I spill tears and his life slips away. His breathing just stops but his nose is filled with heat. His chest is not moving and it makes no sense. The vet returns. 'Do you want to keep his collar?' she asks gently. I stare at her blankly because there is no time for me to have the slightest clue.

I return to the house in a dogless daze. 'Where is Pappy?' says Simon. I mouth words but the shock makes it sound functional. 'You killed my dog,' he says. 'You killed my dog without asking me. How could you? How could you do such a bad thing? How could you do this?' Crushing words continue to crowd his computer screen. I plead and cry but he can't see that I did it for love. 'You are sick. You are unstable,' he says and a howl rises out of me in pure primal anguish. I can't kick him, so I kick his bed instead, as I wail and beg for him to stop.

One sad dog story could be enough to shake down a marriage. Companionship is an angry glare through plate glass windows. We're divided in two different worlds. Where does my husband live and what is it like there? No doubt it is lonely for him too. Oh, how lonely his world must be. Maybe all marriages end up this way. Great love turns to great annoyance.

*

It is a perfect day for a swim but I've got the fear and may need a push. Aifric has returned to her job as an architect and has less time for swims. Michelle is still in full combat with steroids. I have just endured a day of weeping as I told each of the children individually that Pappy is gone. We couldn't make his skin better and the vet had to put him to sleep. Hunter, my little wolf cub, takes it the hardest. Their first giant loss is completely my fault. I can still see the tears dripping from my fingertips into his warm dead fur. I stand on my own at the cove steps, the full weight of dog murder in my bones. I don't think a dive will save me. I may sink like a stone. My husband hates me and I have never felt so alone.

Holidays

'Is France open yet?' asks Sadie every day for three months.
No, pet, it's still closed, but our holiday is unleashed very soon.
I am running away for real this time with the children and
my youngest brother Joe. We are hightailing it to France on
a car ferry to go camping for three weeks without Simon.

I know that we all need this. Since Pappy died, everything
about our home buzzes around my brain like fruit flies that I
can't quite swat away. They've crawled into the bread and
linger on rotten bananas. Our house has the hum of a stinky
compost bin, making it impossible to breathe deeply. I feel
just as rotten. I need something, anything to take this buzzing
out of my head and distract me from a cracked chest and my
broken heart. Oh Lord, pour the wine.

I plonk the kids in front of the TV with our carer Anna
and sneak out to the cove. It can't work this time. I am too
far gone and the tide won't be right. The tide is perfect. I leave

a small pile of clothes on the rocks. My mind is relaxing as soon as I smell the air and my feet touch rock. Cold sea can blow those flies away in one SWOOSH! Three dives later I know that real magic is here. The stones hold secrets and the dread in my heart floats free. It is all so solitary and dreamlike I wonder if it is real. Twenty minutes later I am back home.

The summer Irish water doesn't even pack enough punch for me these days. I'm beginning to believe that prolonged happiness is some sort of bullshit. Intense beautiful living involves pain. I know you, pain, my old buddy, we have been friends for so long now, what would I do without you? Life would be bright and shiny, lacking complex cloud shapes. Steeped in blue skies and anaesthesia, I could become a bored drunk with brown skin. For now I'd much rather dip my toes in cold water and plunge.

Maybe some day life won't be so busy. Pain will lift and I might miss it. Expect quiet days by the lake with a chick-lit novel. I can't quite imagine it. Where would I be without the dark, raging waves and the torture? Maybe nowhere good.

Simon insists on getting Pappy cremated. He is returned to me condensed into a cardboard cylinder printed with lush green leaves. I am not ready to show this to anyone, so I panic. I shove him under the passenger seat of my car and bring him to France. Pappy always loved a long car journey.

Holidays are a funny old game. Expect the unexpected. You expect that you will relax. You don't expect to be driving like a maniac, hundreds of miles on French and Spanish motorways where the speed limit is 130 kilometres and you're clocking 150 and 160 on those sweet French hills.

Fresh off the ferry, I wobble nervously on the right and overtake with a shudder. This translates rather quickly into DON'T FUCK WITH ME PEOPLE AND GET OUT OF MY WAY. Someone is clearly chasing me. Who is chasing me? Don't look over your shoulder because Joe is blocking the mirror with the map and you might get sideswiped by a zippy Renault Clio weaving in and out of lanes. French drivers don't seem to indicate.

We drive through mountains into Spain. These borders are free. I had half hoped for the danger of dogs, guns or at least barbed wire. Lovely roads fly high up on stilts through the Pyrenees. Look, children! *Look* at the view! Heads in books don't even look up and Uncle Joe is asleep.

The Costa Brava is awesomely lawless. We don't give a shit. *De nada* – have another beer, wear your shoes around the pool, carry chips and chilled sangria to your deckchair, push each other down the water-slide, do a flippin' backflip if you're able – the lifeguard is smiling and really doesn't care.

A dwarf dressed in a giant sun costume is the campsite mascot. The short-legged sunshine dances through tall, hot girls, pushing kids into the pool. Whatever, *de nada*, we drink lots of cheap beer and smoke sneaky fags because they are criminally cheap. This is all a bit nasty and fun and so very friendly. The Spanish seem to love kids spontaneously. Waiters make beds out of chairs for the twins when they fall asleep at midnight dinners. We eat at the Mini Golf Restaurant. As the name suggests, this is total tourist heaven.

Someone is still chasing me. I can't relax or sleep at night. The cheesy love songs at the pool area go on all day and, oh Jesus, could someone just change this music to something dancy and empty of emotional Cheddar? Eyes are welling up here. My chin is trembling and I might just cry in a sun-soaked bikini, lip-synching the words to Whitney Houston. Simon sends me the odd functional email and it's out of tune with the Cheddar.

Relax gear begins to ease in. We go to Barcelona for a day. Barcelona is a magical place so obviously we go straight to McDonald's. Children are thirsty. Then we get on an open-top tour bus and plug in headphones for two hours. We drive around with mystery tour sunstroke, looking at this gorgeous land. The buildings are spellbinding. Arden leans over the bus, loses his hat and cries for a long time. His face looks crushed and squinty in the sun. The twins pass out and wake up cross and sweaty. We unstick our legs from the seats, leave imprints of our asses for all time, get off the bus and drag little legs to a train ride home.

There is a water-slide park. Jack begs to do the freefall with Uncle Joe, and I might puke with the motherly stress. We wave to distant dots, before they plummet together from up high. Jack survives and cackles at the bottom with a wide open grin. Subdued Uncle Joe has a tanned face alarmingly drained to grey ash. Holiday spells are being woven and we hold them in our bronzed, sticky hands. You can't take that away from me, Whitney Houston.

Why is sorrow sitting beside me in this sunny place with no shadows? I hadn't realised how much my home life hurt. The extent of the battering has left large bruises. The muscles in my neck scream and spasm at night when I wake drenched in raw anxiety. Tension tails me to the pool, nudges me at dinner and asks me to dance when the lights are turned out. I lie in my narrow camp bed, tossing in sweaty sheets. Holiday, I have yearned for you for so long. What cruel trick is this?

We follow the coast road over winding cliffs to a tinier town called Tossa de Mar. Old buildings and ruins cut into the cliffside. The horizon leads us to a beautiful beach with bobbing speedboats. All seven of us march through hot sand and plunge into the ocean. I crawl out and lie on the sand. My toes dig deep. Arden collects Spanish sea glass and silently deposits pieces on my sunbathing tummy. The sea works its usual magic and I find peace. Holiday, there you are, so nice to meet you.

We drive back to France and someone is chasing me again. The French may be stricter but their food is a cosmic explosion.

The campsite is run like a military base dressed up in sparkly drag. Have fun but don't break the rules and don't you dare wear dirty shoes by the pool.

It turns out that after you make your escape from one coast to another, drive the length of France to dip in the Mediterranean, you feel powerful briefly, then just lonely again. The big world out there can be much bigger and lonelier and you are harder to decipher out of context. I am a sunburnt blip in a congregation of tanned couples and F cars.

People we meet naturally presume that Joe is my husband. Joe is eight years younger than me so I am tickled. Poor Joe cannot hide the absolute horror from his face. We talk about getting him a T-shirt that says 'I'm just the fun uncle', or perhaps, 'They're not mine'.

Joe is such easy company, he brings me back to my roots and normalises me in a good way. I struggle through his boring footballer biography and he steals my *Game of Thrones*. We share tasks and he shoulders small children, with a special place for Sadie, his doting god-daughter. There are few people who would actually look forward to a holiday with this circus. The kids and I know we are very lucky.

For a married couple, Joe and I look remarkably like brother and sister. This sparks fun driving conversations about couples who are clones of each other and dogs that look like their owners. 'Don't mention dogs,' I hiss. 'I miss Pappy!'

wails Hunter on cue from the back. 'He's closer than you think,' I sigh. 'What do you mean?' Joe pounces and then his face drops. 'Is he here?' I smile and Joe's eyes narrow. 'He's under my seat, isn't he?' he says, deadpan. I shrug and then struggle to keep the wheel straight as Joe hops around like he's on an anthill. The kids are too distracted by comic books and Hunter's wailing to grasp our frantic giggles.

We relish long laughs, drink fine wine and get cleaner in France doing drenched runs in the 36 degree heat. Mont Saint-Michel is another enchanted place; we stop there on the way home. From afar, it's a pop–up-book pointy island over flat Normandy lands. We approach from a distance humming the 'Ivory Tower' film score from *The NeverEnding Story*. In close range, cross-faced army guys with guns are patrolling it and the tour bus driver screams at Hunter for standing in the luggage bay. He tries to ram a tourist car in front that dared to overtake him. I love angry French people.

On the overnight ferry home we attack the all-you-can-eat buffet, dance and watch a magician climb into a giant man-sized balloon. He takes Joe's shoe and pours a drink into it, in the shittest magic trick of all time. We clap with joy until our hands hurt.

Back home, someone is still chasing me. Who is it? Oh hello, old friend, it's only you, loneliness. I can see your shape again now we're clear of all that sunshine. You had me worried there, in a stalker kind of way, but that's OK. I suppose I can handle your prowling. There are bigger things to worry about.

Our holiday has put us out of synch with Simon. Family and nurses have forgotten how to coordinate in the same space. Simon lights up to see the kids and they snuggle their tanned skin around him. Words typed to me are still frugal and his eyes glare with disdain. We seem to lose so many Saturdays. Kids grapple with boredom and bounce off walls, waiting for Simon to get up. He emerges in crisp trousers and shirt to say he doesn't want to go anywhere. Rejected and lonely, I bundle the kids up to take them to the cove. I miss Uncle Joe.

Some days just feel like you are failing spectacularly. Running away is supposed to save a day. Tears fall on rocks and I brush them out of sight from summer bathers and lounging families. The cove is always a safe place for such things, but today trouble is brewing between brothers.

Arden and Jack exchange cross words. Stones get thrown at close range. One stone hits its target straight in the neck. Scuffles and blood-curdling screams entertain a busy summer beach. Jack is the man with the winning aim. 'Go to the car,' I scold and he storms off the beach. We follow a few minutes later and Jack is nowhere to be found.

We drive around Greystones, with Arden hanging his

head out the window like an anxious puppy. Is that him on the rocks? No, he was wearing jeans. 'We should call the police, Momma, maybe he's been kidnapped,' pipes up Raife. We drive around for half an hour, circling the same path. On the third round we see him standing white-faced on the corner. I beep the horn and he looks up, haunted. A chalky ghost runs towards us and gets in the car.

Jack had been hiding on the adjacent beach and got a fright when the car was gone. My boy had run away for real. 'Never do that again,' I gasp, hugging him close. 'I won't,' he muffles from somewhere deep within my armpit. I believe him, more than I believe myself. I love to run, but sometimes my family needs me to stay still. I can't stay still long enough for Simon, but I have to try. The kids miss their Uncle Joe too and I should pay attention.

I am totally prepared for stillness. I will settle into couch cushions and put the kettle on. This is easy because something wonderful has happened. My parched and shrivelled plants shudder their collective relief. Marian has come back to work, fighting fit and with smiling eyes. Orchids will bloom in her honour and we can spread into some kind of home again. I want to hug her tightly and never let go. Be gentle with those newly healed bones. 'What about that moon swim, Ruth?' asks Marian with a mischievous grin.

War Wounds

Marian and I just cannot sit still. We are hopping around on our moon-dancing feet. 'Let me check my moon calendar,' Marian announces like a mystic wizard. Expert fingers swipe her touchscreen tablet, gleaning moon data. 'The Harvest Moon is on 16 September this year,' she reads. Well of course it is. I chuckle in disbelief. My head-shaking puts Marian on high alert. 'What? *What*?' she demands. 'Simon and I got married on 16 September. It's our wedding anniversary,' I explain. There is dumbfounded silence. Screams follow that frighten small children. I make breathless phone calls to the Tragic Wives. Rise up, ladies. The full moon swim is on.

I can't sleep at night. If you're no longer afraid of the dark, then maybe days get easier. The moon holds mysteries to agitate the most anxious souls. Let's night swim, embrace the dark, dive into black velvet and get drunk on infinity.

*

The cove in September is a busy spot. Warm days mean crowds stick around for longer. Rocks are thronged with summer stragglers eating chips. We elbow our way down the steps and plunge in beside plucky teenagers. They ignore us and leap off rocks, shouting big words over one another.

Evening is a quieter time to swim, even though our club numbers are growing. With a miniature Pomeranian cradled close, Yasmin skips her way into our hearts. She sets her beatbox to some funky tunes on the rocks and braves the water with charming enthusiasm. The dog is so tiny he waits quivering on a lead attached to her handbag. Maire from Sligo shames me with her fearlessness. 'Those aren't big waves,' she scoffs, as we wade in from the shore to get hammered and rolled repeatedly.

Aifric returns one day with fierce sea-hungry eyes. 'Everything is so busy,' she gasps, 'I need to swim.' Mornings find her peeling off smart clothes to dive in before hitting the office. She admits to sneaky post-swim licks of her arm behind her computer monitor. Mermaid arms taste salty. It's an all-day reminder of that magic first dip.

There're still a couple of weeks to go before the full moon swim, but I bundle the five kids into the car. They're in their pyjamas under warm hoodies. We spin down to the cove as dusk is falling. Michelle is there, steroid-free and healed, glowing brown and golden. A bearded Galen sits in his wheelchair flanking the railings, as close as he can get to the sea. Bodhi cuddles in on his knee. Aifric is here with warm rugs and tea. Random friends out walking stop to chat, and suddenly there is a gathering. This is the Michelle and Galen effect. They are people gatherers wherever they go.

Ladies climb down seaweed-stained rocks because the tide is too far out for step swimming. Some daughters get in too, while their brothers wave sticks and slide off distant sand dunes. Sadie stands on the steps with baffled arms outstretched and roars, 'Why are only the LADIES in the water?' 'Because it's Ladies' Cove and we're *mermaids*,' we laugh. There is whooping and panting as we tread water between chats. The boys get jealous and join in. We scramble over slimy rocks to dive again and again. Galen throws a stick repeatedly for Casper the wonderdog who whines and retrieves it. The dog climbs rocks better than all of us.

It is so glorious we stay in much longer than we should. Eventually, I clamber out over sharp rocks, with the sea shakes and seaweed in my fingernails. I hop up to my car on wet feet. I return with a pocket first-aid kit. Plasters are passed around for bleeding toes, knuckles, elbows and knees. Aifric's teacup moves through so many shaky hands, most of the tea slops over the rim. We laugh with faces open, eyes bright and heads emptied. Night has fallen fully by the time I get the windswept children back in the car and drive home to bed with headlights on.

We are now swimming twice a day and we crave danger.

Michelle visits our smiling hairdresser, who wonders what on earth all this green stuff is in her hair. We get closer than ever to becoming fully fledged mermaids. If the tide is out we scale rocks to dive. Crawling back out, our toes hook into barnacled rock crevices. Strands of seaweed tickle our knees and waves slam our backs as we rise out of the water. Our numb bodies get scuffed and scraped and that is good. Macabre blood runs off limbs and it is painless because of the cold. 'This is badass,' I say, as I count my bloody war wounds. Hours later, the cuts that looked so dramatic reveal themselves, bashfully, to be mere tiny scrapes.

The week prior to 16 September, the moon teases us with an increasingly curvier shape. The 14th is the anniversary of Galen's accident. Friends gather that morning at the harbour with him to swim again. This year Michelle gets in the water too. Galen slips into the sea and rolls on to his back with outstretched arms. I watch him survey an expanse of sky and his mouth opens wide with laughter. His face has floated right up out of pain's reach. He looks weightless with a mad, happy head.

My throat grows a lump as I watch Michelle and Galen swim together. I tread water because I want to stay in the sea as long as Galen does. Stubbornness almost freezes me because he doesn't want to get out. This amphibian nutter will turn me into a blue-lipped Smurf. I don't believe we are just numbing ourselves in this sea. I look at my friends coping and surviving. Like the rolling of waves, the thrill of the dive, the rush of cold, they choose to stay unchained. This is as free as we can all possibly be.

Michelle returns to the harbour that night, with Yasmin and their collective children. I catch them between football pickups and it's another party. Bodhi runs up and down the slipway, a naked boomerang that never wants to stop. The moon isn't full yet, but it looks so close. The harbour has become a giant bath, lit by a glorious round globe. A large seal pops his head up close by. 'We've named him Ron,' giggles Michelle's daughter. Seals look cute but I don't know how I feel about swimming with one. We screech and splash and float on our backs howling at the big yellow moon 'AAAAAAAAOOOOOOHHHHHH!' It is the perfect evening; if only the harbourmaster would give us a chase.

Swims like this clean the cobwebs from my mind, like clearing the laundry basket with a good run of hot washes. I am a woman restored. Happy washing is something perhaps only housewife brains can understand. Housewife is a word that is mostly outdated. I struggle with the title when filling out forms. My pen scrawls around Lady of the House, Maker of Homes, Home Engineer, Family Manager, Homestead Economist, Mistress of Four Walls, Dreamer of Dreams. I scribble them all out.

Most of these routines that fill my day bore me so much. Cooking is kind of OK, but cleaning makes me shrink. I used to turn on daytime radio to drown out my own soul. Smooth over the silence of a wasted life. I tried reading the newspaper. Tapping into that social hum hurt my ears. I'd rather blow up than blend in.

I keep looking in the mirror, staring at myself because I am shocked by the person I see. She is so much herself, more herself than herself could be. Moon swimming makes her wild-eyed with excitement. There is power in doing exactly what you should be doing. Call me anything you like. I want to sing my own tune. The moon and the ocean are calling me.

Moon Swim

'Happy Anniversary,' I say to Simon with my usual morning kiss to his forehead. 'Can you sit with the kids tonight while the girls and I go for a naked full moon swim?' We have run ourselves ragged together for so long. Now I need this moon swim to save myself. The smile in his eyes gives me hope he understands that. I'm still not sure. He might just be enjoying my gift of a mental image composed of all-girl nakedness.

I hum around the house all day, dreaming of full moons. I can taste the thrill of shy bodies standing naked over a dark sea. Our birth scars, broken veins and secret wobbly bits will bask in moonlight. We can defy our brains and dive deep with hammering hearts. The moment feet find water, bodies will work against worried brains. We'll leap and mainline right into the pulse of nature. There is so much fear around illness, and this is the opposite of that. I am terrified.

Daydreams get slightly altered at the school gates. I whisper my plans to a friend. 'You're getting naked at the cove ... *tonight*?' she cries. I nod and grin. 'But, Ruth? It's Culture Night in Greystones. There's an outdoor cinema on the beach tonight. It'll be packed. With hundreds! They're screening *Jaws*.'

'Holy shit!' I bark within earshot of little people. I clasp hand to mouth as swarms of tiny faces glance up. We are doubled over with laughter. 'Holy shit,' I repeat quietly in a more school-friendly tone. Tragic Wives should clearly pay more attention to the social calendar.

As daylight fades, I leave the kids cuddled up in bed, with Simon, watching a movie together. I might see a movie too, I wink, waving them all goodbye. 'Good luck, Momma,' they cheer, with popcorn-stuffed cheeks.

The cove throbs with a carnival atmosphere. Food stalls blast out the heat of roast chicken on spits and hot barbecue sauce. A large cinema screen hangs facing the sea and coloured deck-chairs are lining up on the shore.

We climb down rocks on the other side of the steps to a small inlet, hidden away from the crowds. Huddled together on our secret beach, wrapped in blankets, we watch the moon rise. I never knew that the moon rose like the sun and feel like a bit of a dumbass. It is large and pure orange. Marian, Aifric, Michelle and I cuddle together like a wolf pack with the wild urge to howl. It is utterly beautiful and I feel total love for these women. Sharing this view with my Tragic Wives feels mightily untragic.

The moon rises high and the light slips away. Darkness falls and the cinema screen begins to flicker. A full carpet of people covers the beach; with their backs to the sea, they watch the screen. We feel detached from these cave dwellers who stare at dancing shapes on a wall. They are lit by the light of the projector, as we lurk on distant steps steeped in shadows. My tribe and I face the light of the moon and we stand over harsh ocean.

I wish I could say we are the wise philosophers of this gathering, but we are closer to wild-eyed lunatics, wishing we were fully naked, only we might get arrested. We have reluctantly settled for skimpy bikinis instead. Cave dwellers keep their backs to us and don't intrude on our space. There is room here for everyone. It feels like they've gathered just for us, filling up the background and willing us to jump.

'Look at the moonpath on the water,' whispers Michelle. 'I want to swim in it.' She has that crazed look in her eye, like if she followed that moonpath she might never come back.

The Tragic Wives' Swimming Club gets some new members for the night. Alison takes photos. Helen hands out towels. Margie is here for the full swim. Marian has never swum from the steps before and is determined this will be her first time. A fully female energy is harnessed on these rocks as we drop our towels.

The water truly looks like black velvet and is teasingly rough. Waves slap up and hit the rusty step railings. We wait until the *Jaws* theme music is playing and then we dive in. Marian makes it all the way down the steps to her waist and gets frozen with fright. 'I can't,' she sobs as I climb out of the water to help her. First time is just too big, wrapped in all this darkness. She has brought herself as far as she can go and I won't push her.

The cold and the moon have silenced us to startled gasps as we plunge, dive and swim circles. 'I hope Ron the seal doesn't get ideas watching *Jaws*,' I giggle, before diving one last time. A group of teenagers, bored by the screen, have drifted towards us. 'You're all fucking mental,' they mutter respectfully. For the moment, they have stopped ignoring us.

We race to the warmth of the pub afterwards for chats and hot whiskeys. Back in the glow of indoors I look around the table at this awesome group of women. I marvel at the ladies I now count as friends. They are brave and honest and we give nothing but love to each other. It is a powerful find of belonging to feel steeped in your own tribe. One-to-one friendship is wonderful but tonight we weave together as a group. It is a night full of real joy and laughter. I feel more content than I can remember in a long time, or else the whiskey has gone straight to my head.

*

Marian is disgusted with herself that she only got halfway in. She insists on meeting me at the cove two days later. Treading water, I coax her with soothing words and hope to God she hurries up before I get hypothermia. She eventually throws herself from the rocks with impressive ear-shattering shrieks. Random onlookers spontaneously clap. She emerges with manic, unfixed eyes. 'It's bloody *freezing*! Where's the fucking adrenaline rush, Ruth?' she hollers, accusingly. '*You liar*!!! I'm still waiting for it to kick in!' I laugh as she screams like some kind of adrenaline-soaked whirling dervish.

I still yearn for that naked swim. Seawater and blood plasma have the same composition, according to Mark, a seasoned Greystones swimmer. He speaks and bends into startling yoga shapes by the cove steps. Man, I just love his hippie science talk. 'The amniotic fluid in the womb is similar to seawater. All that iodine is so good for you too,' he adds, before diving in with dolphin perfection. He has disappeared into the deep. We can wait minutes before he comes back up again for air.

Our naked full moon moment happens two months later, on 14 November. It's an unseasonable warm night and no one else is around. The moon hides behind clouds and three of us hide under towels. There is an awkward pause. 'Who will be the first to ... ?' I wonder, but Aifric has already strolled by me, a casual naked goddess. Wow. I follow her bum cheeks down the steps into the black waters. Maire is right behind me. We stand in a line as the wind whips naked parts. I screech and dive in.

Skinny dipping is the ultimate caress from nature, Marian once said, and that's exactly what it feels like. I have never felt so silky. Mother of God and Earth and Sea, I can only gasp at the feeling. I am not me, I am part of the water. It surrounds every part of me. We dive and pant and climb until the cold is done with us.

Maybe this is some kind of death wish or my sorry soul drawn to eternity. I don't really know. My mortal coil is unravelling under the wild moon, in an inky mass of cold water. When I swim like this I am fearless. A mad moonpath is leading me towards better dreams. But the more I breathe in time to the ocean, the more Simon and I seem to be out of synch.

'I'd do that again', says Aifric softly. 'The 14 of December is the next full moon,' smiles Maire. Hello to a chilly Happy Christmas. Getting dressed, we talk calmly about swims and moonbows. Moonbows are like rainbows, says Maire, made by water and moonlight instead of the sun. It's difficult for the human eye to discern colours in a moonbow so they appear white. Moonbows are rare but they do happen. I feel calm and sleepy. There is no wild elation here. Just deep satisfaction. I go home and sleep deeply for the first time in years.

Waves (and Cheese Puffs)

Storms are provoking the sea to wild heights. Cars swing up past the harbour and slow down in shock at the sheer sight of these enormous waves. A swim in this would spit you out for life. Passers-by stand transfixed, like aliens have just landed. Crashing waves are by far my favourite. These waves are so intense they move in fast-forward motion. They are badass fuckers that chomp on the cove steps in big bites. Swarming over land and rock, they make everything look tiny. Carried by the wind they seem to be in the very air we breathe. Onlookers gasp for breath, knowing this sea is strong enough to bring the whole world down, bang after glorious bang.

For a whole week, the massive waves consume the coastline. White chunks of foam blow from the sea and land on the road like snow. Water sprays on car windows leaving salty snail trails. When the waves finally settle, a new set of steps

has appeared at Greystones South Beach. The sea just exca-
vated them like some swift, furious, archaeological dig. 'Where
did the steps come from?' ask the kids. 'Those steps got buried
years ago,' explains Phil, our Greystones native. 'It's an old
swimming spot that used to be called The Men's'. Alleluia and
peace on earth. The men just got their steps back. Ladies' Cove
is now truly mine.

Sadie runs roaring into the kitchen in dramatic floods of tears.
'My heart is in tiny pieces!' she wails. 'Raife just smashed my
heart.'

'I wouldn't give her the remote control,' explains Raife,
rolling his eyes. I want to tell Sadie that hearts can survive in
pieces. I have only ever risked my heart for something that is
worthwhile, so smash away. Remote controls may not count
as worthy, so maybe I'll wait till she's older. If Arden keeps
gathering sea glass from the beach, my heart pieces can survive
like this indefinitely. I rattle his growing collection around in
my coin purse. Sometimes it spills on to tabletops as I count
out sea glass in busy coffee shops. Pappy still resides under
the passenger seat of the car. I think he belongs there now.

'When I first came here you used to hoover the house every
morning at 7 a.m.,' Marian reminds me. Sweet Jesus, we're well
rid of that manic lady. The superhero costume slipped for
good reason. Weeds may choke the shrubs, dust can gather
in corners, toilets crust over with wayward boy streams. The

housewife will get to all of it eventually, but for now there are important chats pending with Marian, over steaming cups of tea.

'Momma, when we grow up we're gonna be mermaids in the sea, just you and me. We'll dive in and jump back out because that's what mermaids do. I want to be a mermaid just like you, Momma. Our magic necklaces will scare away the sharks, won't they?'

'Of course they will, Sadie,' I reply. Hunter whines in protest. 'I want to be a dog,' he grumbles, 'but dogs can't swim underwater.' His chubby face wobbles in a thinking moment. 'I'm gonna be a mermaid dog,' he decides with faraway eyes.

Raife marches into the kitchen with a notepad tucked under his arm. 'Momma, give me one of those tablets for greasing up your brain, quick!' he demands. 'You mean . . . a fish oil tablet?' I guess, at a reach. 'That's the one. I want to write a book the same as you and Dadda, so I need a greasy brain,' he says. Lord help us, another writer, I think. At least he's given up on the limp.

Days are getting colder so I light the stove and cook baked potatoes. I'm being good to myself because a half-made-up rhyme is playing in my head. *Remember, remember, this day in November. Give us a break MND, for my marriage's sake. If you won't give me one, I'll take two, the better for us, and the worse for you.* Perched on the noisy bed beside Simon and plumped up with cushions, we watch the first assembly of his film, *My Name is Emily*. We are beyond dead dogs, distant beds and suspicious glances, and we share a moment. This film spans our entire marriage. So many of Simon's thoughts and philosophies sing through it. I can see him clearly, a cheeky boy with a charming grin, driving cars too fast.

The sorrow that's deep in me rises up and overwhelms my body. Tears pour out. Huge arms of grief wrap around the years and squeeze them in close. In this moment, I love Simon so much. I cling to his Tin Man chest that moves mechanically and I hang there like a soggy rag. Simon cries too. It is the first thing we have shared in such a long time and that makes me cry harder.

This life is so comical. Strangers fill kettles in our kitchen and scuffle around with cups. It is comical and cruel, yet I still hold on to my husband's magnificent heart. A tender glance later and this moment will be gone, but I won't forget.

Jack has gone quiet again. 'I wish Dadda didn't have MND,' he says for the hundredth time. 'Me too, it's shit, Jack,' is my reply. I stare at him carefully. Looking at our handsome boy with a heavy, worried, head, I wonder whether that head ever looked any way lighter. 'But you know what?' I add, 'Thank God for cheese puffs. Crispy, cheesy goodness crunching around your mouth. I'm so glad they exist. I mean, imagine a world without cheese puffs?' I wave arms for dramatic effect.

Jack's face lights up and he grins the cheesiest grin. He really does like cheese puffs very much. 'Yeah,' he beams. We will always have cheese puffs, Jack. ALWAYS.

I go to bed that night and have the freakiest dream. A large gypsy man in a bowler hat is holding a tray full of bowls. 'Put money in the bowl to get healed,' he shouts. I'm contemplating which bowl to pick when I notice Simon's parents sitting beside a blanket. What's under there? I wonder. I lift up the blanket and Simon is underneath. 'We cured him with the right bowl,' they say. His tracheostomy is gone but he is pale and breathless and young in the face like our wedding photo. 'Why didn't you tell me?' I cry, and I am really cross at them for leaving me out. 'If he's cured he needs fresh air to breathe!' I panic, grabbing him and weeping now with relief.

Simon and I run from blankets and bowls to a wide-open field where crowds of people are dancing all around us. We are kissing each other and laughing and then kissing everyone else with huge hugs. Our love has stretched out past the boundaries of each other and we are bonded to all these other people too. A bearded midget randomly walks by and I don't know why except that small people are magical beings who always seem to wander for no reason into other people's dreams. I wake up feeling baffled but calm and alarmingly carefree.

*

A large moon lingers, with a streak of white streaming out from one side. I think I've just seen my first moonbow, but I'm not sure, so I don't mention it. Arden comes home from school the next day saying, 'Jack Diamond told Teacher he saw a moonbow last night. What's a moonbow, Momma?' Moonbows are rare but they do happen. Maybe I'll go moonbow hunting with the tribe when we brave our next naked full moon swim.

Marian has brought her piano keyboard to work and sits playing *The Snowman* theme, with fast-moving fingers. The children and I dance slowly around the kitchen, because her playing is really good. 'We're walking in the air!' Sadie warbles along. Marian laughs and it feels like family.

I stop to survey the circus around me. Simon sits by the fire and lets me cut his nails. Children are dancing. Daydreams these days swirl closer to real hopes. I hope the waves get calmer at the cove soon. I hope that ladies congregate by chance at the steps, within minutes of each other, clutching towels straight after the school run. The Bagpipe Man might be walking the wall, serenading the sea and dogs will run. Ron the seal may pop his head up for a glance.

I know I can be brave as long as the waves keep pounding. That's just what waves do. I hope Simon and I can be kind to one another. The landscape may change, but it is always surprising and beautiful. This is great love after all and that's just what love does too.

'Momma, do you like swimming ... SO MUCH?!' lisps Hunter from the back seat of the car. 'Of course she does,' replies Raife. 'It's her hippie hobby'. I'm no hippie and it's not a hobby, I grin, this is everything. I'll keep flashing Madame Moon for ever, as long as she shows that full frontal. It's a new rhythm that's old as time. I follow the tides and the moon. If we can grab some of that moonpath, I won't hesitate. Just dive right in. Like the waves themselves, don't you dare mess with me. I am free.

Acknowledgements

Aifric Aiken and Michelle Griffin, I've said enough nice things about both of you but thanks for putting up with a friend who insists on writing about her friends. She did *what?* Such a *bitch*.

Our superheroes in Australia: Cath, Daragh and Theo Monaghan. Phones are crap but you all sing loudly in my soul every day; probably some warbly indie-girl song that Cath and Simon would love.

Matt and Mary Darby, I will always want to be like you.

Phil 'Six-pack' McDarby, a gifted human in so many ways, it is shocking. Don't ever stop making me laugh, even when I beg and weep 'please' from a foetal position on the floor.

Galen English, the ridiculously good-looking car battery who also has really good-looking children. You rock.

Marian 'Angel' Condron, the universe is infinitely better with you in it, so please drive carefully.

Mick 'Moonhead' Minogue, it makes me happy that you exist. I wrote this book to impress you.

Kathryn Kennedy and Frankie Fenton, if it wasn't for you I never would have met . . . no, wait, that's your story not mine. Giant lovehearts to both of you. Don't call the baby Emily, even if it's a girl. Along with Lesley McKimm, mad stuff happens when you lot are around. I've learned to just go with it.

Paula 'Amazon' Cousins, you carried Simon to a place I couldn't. You would also definitely win at arm wrestling. I will always be grateful.

Some Cove specials: awesome and epic Diamond brothers Sean and Jack, gorgeous Holly Doyle, Anita and Soren Griffin, Maire Giblin, Margie Desmond, Helen Coughlan, Yasmin Fortune, sea glass lady Nancy Falkow McBride, seaweed gentleman Mark Lawlor.

Yvonne Leon and Treasa Gibney, lucky me, I get to call you both friends.

The Happy Pear Cafe, the groovy heart of Greystones.

Roisin Ingle, you put me in the *Irish Times* in my swimsuit. How did that happen? You are the finest person and writer, with a heart to match.

Sarah 'Canadian badass' Williams from the Sophie Hicks Agency, my agent with the best sense of humour, you always just got it.

Clara Farmer from Chatto & Windus, I am so very relieved that you were the one to help me write this book. And Charlotte Humphery, your eloquence made the editing process entirely pain free.

Emma Norton, Jennie Scanlon and Chelsea Morgan

Hoffmann from Element Pictures, three amazing women and many adventures ahead.

Alison McKenny, if you lived in Greystones we would totally make you swim.

My long suffering parents, Pat and Dave 'What did you say about us now?' O'Neill. Sorry, but it's all your fault.

Catherine O'Neill, thank God I have a sister who is no one else but you.

My brother Joe O'Neill, the kids and I would lock you up in a box and keep you in our kitchen forever if we could. I don't care if that sounds creepy.

The other brothers, John, David and Michael O'Neill, board games without you are just not the same.

My dear husband, Simon Fitzmaurice. 'It's fucking mental being stuck inside your head Ruth, I got freaked out and had to stop reading'; your compliment made me swoon.

All the *sportos, motorheads, geeks, sluts, bloods, wastoids, dweebies and dickheads* who have ever graced our doorstep, I adore you; I think you are all *righteous dudes*.

Our collective tribe of children: Sofia, Ava and Isobel McDarby; Kai, Tasiana, Levi and Bodhi Griffin English; Jack, Raife, Arden, Sadie and Hunter Fitzmaurice. What a merry band of heart-punching, ass-kicking laughter monsters. I hope you never ever become real life respectable adults. Did I say that out loud?

Thank you all and sorry if I ever made you cry.